Inner Tantric Yoga
Working with the Universal Shakti
Secrets of Mantras, Deities and Meditation

By David Frawley

LOTUS
PRESS

TWIN LAKES, WISCONSIN, USA

COMPOSITION/LAYOUT: Trice Atkinson

COVER ART: Hinduism Today Magazine

LINE DRAWINGS: Kanika Tripathi

COPY EDITING: Margo Bachman

Printed in the United States of America

Library of Congress Cataloging-in-Publication Data: 2008921059

ISBN: 978-0-9406-7650-3

Published by:
Lotus Press, P.O. Box 325, Twin Lakes, Wisconsin 53181 USA
web: www.lotuspress.com
e-mail: lotuspress@lotuspress.com
800-824-6396

Table of Contents

Foreword

Yoga is such a big part of Western culture these days that most of us believe we're already aware of everything it has to offer. After all, Hatha Yoga classes are available everywhere people exercise together, and yogic stress reduction techniques are taught at medical clinics around the country. Everyone knows how healthy a vegetarian diet is, and that meditation produces an impressive array of psychological and physiological benefits. This resume is dazzling enough; what more could there be?

Plenty, it turns out. In fact the more time I spend with traditionally trained yogis and yoginis from India, the more amazed I am at how little of the authentic tradition has reached our shores. It's as if the yoga masters feed us small pieces of it at a time, as much as people raised in our far more materialistic culture are able to assimilate. Only after we've had a chance to digest those teachings do they reveal more advanced techniques and insights.

Looking back, it's easy to see that yoga swept into Western culture in waves. In 1893 Swami Vivekananda first introduced Americans and Europeans to the four great paths: Raja Yoga (physical and mental exercises), Jnana Yoga (the intellectual quest for spiritual experience), Bhakti Yoga (devotion) and Karma Yoga (the practical yoga of enlightened daily activity). In the 1930s Paramahamsa Yogananda initiated Western students into Kriya Yoga, which focused on subtle inner experiences involving the gradual arousal of Kundalini. But it was in the late 1960s that yoga leapt from the fringes of American culture into the mainstream when, thanks to adepts like Maharishi Mahesh Yogi and Swami Rama, claims about yoga's astounding physical effects were finally validated in scientific research studies. Then in the late 1980s

India's yoginis (female yogis) began making their mark here, often emphasizing the spiritual value of social service.

But what is the next wave? Important elements of the yoga tradition—elements considered absolutely essential by most practitioners in India—remain virtually unknown in the West. Ironically, this was not always the case. Historians of Western religious traditions have shown that some of these elements were known to the ancient Greeks and Romans, and were even embraced by many early Christians. Tragically, during the Dark Ages a great deal of spiritual lore disappeared in Europe. The long lost "wisdom of the ancients" was preserved in India however, and beckons us to reclaim it. Are we ready for even deeper and more powerful dimensions of yoga practice?

Most of us first get involved with yoga not because we want to be enlightened but because we want to be healthy. We're got our hands full dealing with the world around us; we don't want to devote hours a day to inner realms when contending with the outside world is challenging enough. We just want to learn some yoga postures and maybe a few tips about cooking healthier meals. But yoga opens the door to inner experience whether we consciously turn the doorknob or not. After an hour of hatha poses and yogic breathing we feel incredible. We're experiencing a level of clarity and tranquility, of focus and well being, that we've rarely touched before. We get to know ourselves in a whole new way, as a calm, bright, creative *soul* rather than a restless, worried, chronically dissatisfied *mind*. Yoga practice has carried us beyond our body and thought processes, and introduced us to *spirit*.

This is the point where many students start exploring yoga philosophy and sign up for meditation classes. We learn a whole new vocabulary for amazing inner states that English doesn't even have words for, but that yoga texts describe in detail. We become eager to experience these extraordinary states ourselves. "Enlightenment" is no longer just an abstraction to us—it becomes an actual goal.

But then, for many yoga students, something goes wrong. As I travel around the United States visiting different yoga centers, students report a common problem: they complain their meditation practice eventually becomes so lifeless, it's difficult to stick with it. They've been taught to sit mechanically counting their mantras as if they were spiritual accountants, or to work with their posture and breath as if yoga was nothing more than a clever way to manipulate their nervous system. No wonder they're bored and uninspired!

It's time for the next wave of yogic wisdom to surge across our shores. There is so much more the masters have to share; if we're ready for this knowledge it will sweep us past the stuck points in our practice to a vastly expanded experience of spirituality. This is the aspect of yoga science that cracks us out of our self-preoccupation and opens our meditation to the universal forces flowing around us and through us. This is the knowledge the adepts in India use to lift and expand their personal practice, to *connect* with the living universe in a way that galvanizes their spiritual life. The secret—openly known throughout India but barely hinted at in the West—is the *Devata*, the inner deities or cosmic powers of yoga.

In the book you now hold in your hands, Dr. David Frawley will introduce you to the *Devatas* that lie at the heart of traditional yogic practice. (You should be aware that Devatas were also recognized by spiritual masters like Socrates, Iamblichus and Proclus in the West centuries ago.) The Devatas are the living intelligence in nature, sparks of spirit that guide and illumine, divine beings we've called "angels" in the West without really understanding what angels are. These are the forces that make mantras, yantras and mandalas come alive, that activate our intuitive powers, and that assist and protect us in the state after death.

In all my years of studying the sacred tradition in India, I've never met a yogi or yogini who wasn't actively engaged with these powerful inner energies. They link us with the many *Shaktis* or powers that govern the physical and subtle worlds. They serve as bridges to higher fields of consciousness.

In one sense Devatas are wholly the hidden powers of our own superconscious mind. In another sense they are independent entities operating outside us. In reality they are rooted in a transcendent realm where the distinctions "inner" and "outer" no longer have any relevance. To practitioners in India, they're the essence of spiritual life.

For thousands of years incorporating the Devatas into one's spiritual practice has made inner discipline a pleasure, transforming meditation from mental drudgery into heartfelt worship. Meditation comes alive when Shakti, the power of consciousness, is activated. This is the next level of practice for serious yoga students, a whole new realm of spiritual experience for intrepid inner explorers.

I'm profoundly grateful to Dr. David Frawley for beginning the complex task of introducing these forces to Western students. For decades he has been sharing the wisdom of the East with the students of the West in language we can all understand. He is one of the most respected Western-born scholar-practitioners of the yogic tradition in India itself. Dr. Frawley is the perfect teacher to instruct us in inner Tantric yoga, sharing the cherished secrets that lead to a richer, fuller spiritual life.

Linda Johnsen
Sonoma, California
March, 2007

Note by Lokesh Chandra

Enclosed in this beautiful book are drops of wisdom from the veins of the visualizations of the modern Rishi Vamadeva Shastri (Dr. David Frawley). In his scintillating flow of lucid cosmic language, he leads our psyche from the stormy sea of Maya into the undifferentiated luminous being of Shiva and Shakti. The cosmic processes of the Divine are integrated within the depths of our own being. He raises our consciousness to the pure bliss of *Sat-chid-ananda*, reminding us of the words of the renowned yoga treatise of *Gheranda Samhita*:

> *Let him find in his heart a broad ocean of nectar,*
> *Within it a beautiful island of gems,*
> *Where the sands are bright golden and sprinkled with jewels.*

The perceptive words of Rishi Vamadeva reflect the subtle sound of Yoga leading to the profoundest knowing. As the yogi tries to hear finer and finer tones, he goes into a depth that invokes an absence of mind and senses to eliminate all external stimuli, in preparation of concentration and meditation. From the physical world of senses called *Bhur-loka*, he ascends to the subtle energy regions of the *Bhuvar-loka*, and then to realms of light or *Svar-loka*. Rishi Vamadeva puts these jewels in our hands, whose radiance bursts into the full bloom of Shiva and Shakti. The two are the *Para Samvit* or Supreme Consciousness that fills all existence. The world is a garment of Shiva and Shakti. The ego and things are but waves provoked by divine necessity. This flux of the universe leaps into pure consciousness, into the crystalline brilliance of Shiva and Shakti. In the secret lotus of the heart is the unfolding of Shiva and Shakti.

The Rishi Vamadeva shows the path to the palin-genesis of the spiritual state that has its origins in the depths of the heart. The *Amrita-ratnavali* says: "The essence of all things resides in our bodies," for without the body we cannot catch the glimmer of the Divine. The psychic life of the individual reflects that of the universe. In the Shaiva and Shakta traditions, two intersecting triangles represent the expanse from the One to the All (triangle with the apex downwards) and of reintegration (triangle with the apex upwards). Vamadeva shows the path to awaken this light that dwells asleep in the psyche. He exhorts us to bloom like a lotus flower, beyond the moment to the eternal. This book is an inspiring calligraphy of the Divine that does not speak words, but brings paths of reflections where we walk inside ourselves, to sketch the Echo, to search the sacred rhyme in the sparkle of life, in the interminable imminence forever beyond.

Rishi Vamadeva presents the multiple facets of Yoga, of symbolism, of the fundamental harmony of the Vedic and Tantric transcendence, and of the vast canvas of other innumerable concepts and practices, in crystal clarity of language that conveys the essence to a layman as much as to a scholar. You can hear in his words the murmurs of Vedic rishis in the shimmer of their Vision, the reflection of yogis, the structuring of philosophers, and gaze at the fountains of visions of sadhakas (practitioners). Inner Yoga lives in his jewel-like words that transcend in their clarity even the exegesis of the great masters of India. To read him is to walk inside ourselves in a thread of illumination that guides our meandering reflections.

Prof. Lokesh Chandra
Padma Bhushan, Former Director of the Indian Council
    of Historical Research and Member of the Rajya Sabha
April 2007
Delhi, India

Author's Preface

Shakti is an important principle, almost a mantra, which has entered into the new spirituality at a global level, and the worldwide resurgence of the worship of the Goddess. Shakti is the prime focus of Tantric Yoga, one of India's greatest traditions, which contains a comprehensive worship of the Goddess through beautiful and profound rituals and meditations. Tantra affords us a direct means to access her power and presence through a tradition that has never lost connection to her grace.

Yet Shakti, like Tantra, is a subject that is commonly misunderstood. Shakti is not simply about sexuality or about the feminine, though it includes these in important ways. Shakti relates to all cosmic energies and the union of all opposites. Shakti represents the awesome and cataclysmic powers of the magical Conscious Universe in which we live, on all levels of matter and mind, nature and spirit, the individual and the collective.

Shakti is ultimately the power of the Absolute or 'Pure Consciousness', what is called *Para-Shiva,* the 'Supreme Shiva' in yogic thought. Shiva is the cosmic masculine principle that compliments Shakti as the cosmic feminine force. So any real examination of Shakti must include an examination of Shiva as well.

The cosmic forces of Shiva and Shakti in turn form the basis for the divine powers or deities that rule over all the different processes within the universe. So any real examination of Shakti must look into the role of these deities as well, the great Gods and Goddesses of the living world.

Inner Tantric Yoga examines Shakti in a broader context as the power of universal awareness. It explores Shakti as the underlying source behind all the forces of nature from physical forces like electromagnetism to spiritual energies like the Kundalini. The book looks at

Shakti from two primary perspectives, from a naturalistic point of view and from the point of view of deeper yogic practices of mantra and meditation. It uncovers the Shaktis at work both in the world of nature and in the higher potentials of consciousness within us.

As its name *Inner Tantric Yoga* indicates, the book is not just a presentation of the outer aspects of Tantra or an academic study of the subject, but aims to instruct serious students in the deeper Tantric tradition of Self-realization through working with Shakti and Shiva. The book reflects the larger and older tradition of Tantra, which includes the teachings of Kashmiri Shaivism, South India's Shaiva Siddhanta, the Advaitic Tantra of the great Vedantic guru Shankara, and the work of the great modern Tantric seer Ganapati Muni. Yet, perhaps uniquely, the book reflects the connections between Tantra and the older Vedic tradition, which most modern studies do not understand. It shows how traditional Tantra relates to Vedic rituals and mantras, and how both similarly work with the powers of nature as forces of higher consciousness.

The goal of the book is to help awaken the Goddess and Her powers within us—to energize the Shakti of our deeper being for the realization of our true nature. Shakti is the real power behind any authentic inner yogic process. It is not we as individuals who control or direct the inner movement of Yoga. All that we personally attempt remains but a mere spark, reflection or ray of light of this more powerful Shakti. To really move forward on our path, we must learn to cooperate with the inner Shakti in its deeper activity, which is to unfold the higher potentials of awareness within us, without obstruction.

Inner Tantric Yoga teaches the inner aspect of Yoga, what one could call the 'inner Yoga', of mantra, meditation, and the quest for the higher Self. As such, the book presents a different view of Yoga than what is popular today, which emphasizes the 'outer Yoga' of asana or Yoga postures. While this 'outer Yoga' has its value; its real purpose is to provide a foundation for the 'inner Yoga', not to be an end-in-itself.

Specifically, the book explains several powerful mantras, not only to the Goddess but also to Shiva. In so doing, it is not setting forth these mantras mechanically, to be repeated superficially to fulfill mere personal desires. It is meant to provide an inner contact with the real energy and meaning of the mantras, so that we can use them in a discriminating and transformative manner.

Only use the mantras indicated with a sattvic (pure) intention to promote healing, harmony and the removal of negativities. Use the mantras along with a sattvic (pure) life-style of clean living, good thoughts and respect for the sacred nature of all life. Make sure to first look at the 'Note on the Chanting of Mantra' in Appendix 2 for more information on this topic.

The book is divided into four sections and an appendix.

- The first section explains Shiva and Shakti as cosmic principles relative to the practice of Inner Tantric Yoga, including the importance of the use of deities (Devatas).
- The second section focuses on Shakti and its many powers in the outer world of nature and the inner world of the psyche, including various methods of 'meditation on Shakti' in the body, mind and world of nature.
- The third section focuses on the forms and personalities of the Goddess, primarily Kali, Sundari, Chhinnamasta and Bhairavi and their worship relative to the chakras and Inner Tantric Yoga, including explaining their mantras.
- The fourth section addresses the deeper practices of Tantric Energy and Vedic Light Yogas, providing keys to understanding the process of Self-realization through the chakras.
- The appendix addresses the issues of tradition and the connection between Vedic, Vedantic, Yoga and Tantric teachings, as well as providing a glossary, bibliography, footnotes and other resource material and information.

The book is based on my personal study and practice of Yoga, Tantra, Veda and Vedanta for more than thirty years. It also reflects my work with Ayurvedic medicine and Vedic astrology, though its concern is not with personal healing but with inner transformation. It is closely related to my previous book, *Tantric Yoga and the Wisdom Goddesses* (1994), and like it reflects the teachings of Kavyakantha Ganapati Muni. Ganapati Muni was the chief disciple of Ramana Maharshi, the renowned Advaitic guru of modern India. However, Ganapati was also probably modern India's greatest Sanskrit writer. Most notably, he mastered the secrets of mantra, Tantra, Shakti, Veda and Vedanta through which he connected the entire Yoga tradition into a single stream of inspiration.

Recently eleven volumes of the Muni's collected Sanskrit works have become available, though without English translation, allowing his works to be preserved. This has occurred through the dedicated service of K. Natesan, who now over ninety years of age, is living proof of the grace of both Ramana and Ganapati. I have been fortunate to have known Natesan for many years, and he has been a great source of encouragement in these studies. I hope that this book encourages further study of Ganapati's work as well.

Finally, I would like to dedicate the book to Shambhavi Chopra who served to draw me back into the realms of Shiva and Devi and has shown me the living reality of the deities in their Himalayan abodes. Those looking for a deeper experiential view of the Inner Tantric Yoga should examine her books.

May the Inner Tantric Yoga connect you to the Supreme Shakti and the Supreme Shiva within your deepest nature!

David Frawley (Vamadeva)
Santa Fe, New Mexico
May 2008

PART ONE

Principles of
Inner Tantric Yoga

Only when Shiva is united to Shakti does he gain the power to create. Otherwise the Lord does not even have the power to stir. O Goddess, as you are worshipped by the Creator, Preserver and Destroyer of the universe, how can a mere mortal who has no merit be able to praise you?

SHANKARACHARYA, A 1

This section introduces the main factors of the Inner Tantric Yoga, including Shakti as the power of the Goddess, Shiva as the Supreme Deity of awareness, the Devatas or Gods and Goddesses as the universal cosmic powers, and the higher realities of Atman and Brahman, the Supreme Self and the Absolute. It includes a deeper examination of what Yoga is and how it works on all aspects of our being.

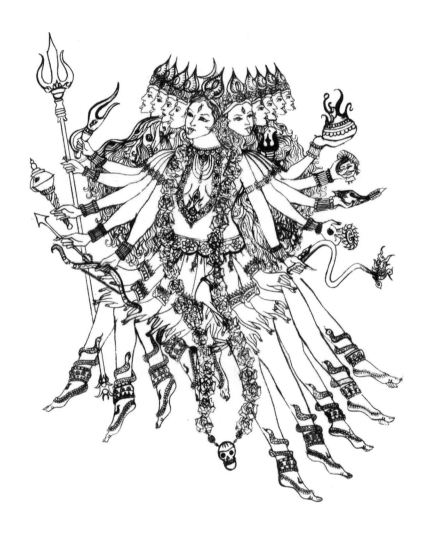

Mahakali

Shakti and Deity Yoga

The art and science of Yoga has a tremendous, if not magical capacity to transform our existence on all levels of body, mind and spirit. It connects us with the awesome forces at the root of the world of nature as well as with the supreme energy that transcends time and space. Performed in the optimal manner, an inner Yoga practice can awaken us to a radically different dimension of awareness in which we can realize all of existence, from the infinitesimal to the infinite, as aspects of our own greater being, consciousness and joy.

For such an inwardly transformative Yoga to be possible, the question inevitably arises: *How can we learn to practically work with the universal forces within us?* Important keys to this inner alchemy lie in the approaches of the ancient Yoga—along both Tantric and Vedic lines—which are largely forgotten or misunderstood in modern Yoga teachings that are usually more physical in nature.

Tantra provides us the understanding of *Shakti* or universal energy necessary for any deep changes to occur within the psyche. Veda provides us with the understanding of *Jyoti* or universal light, to illumine our path beyond the darkness of spiritual ignorance.

Tantric and Vedic Yogas—particularly if used together—enable us to harness the deeper powers of Yoga in an experiential manner, just as modern science shows us how to use the subtle natural forces of electricity or solar power for our technological benefit.

However, to really work with the inner powers of Yoga, we must first be willing to live a life of experiential spirituality. True Yoga practice is not just a hobby, sidelight, exercise system or a business. For this to occur, our daily activities must become part of a deeper ritual, offering and meditation to the great Unknown. We must consecrate all aspects of our being to the inner force and the inner light deep within us.

We must dedicate ourselves to the 'Inner Yoga' or *Antar Yoga* in Sanskrit,[1] the union with the divine energies within ourselves that has always been the essence of real Yoga, not simply to the physical or psychological aspects of Yoga that have so far predominated in the modern world, what is more appropriately called the 'Outer Yoga' or *Bahir Yoga* in Sanskrit. It is in the direction of this ancient and transformative inner Yoga that the journey of this book proceeds.

Classical Yoga and Self-Realization

We are all seeking a greater Self-realization, trying to unfold our hidden potentials in one way or another, gradually moving towards a more expansive energy and awareness. Yet we seldom examine the nature of the Self that we are seeking and how it relates to the greater existence around us. Only if we discover our deepest Self and spiritual essence, can we find lasting peace and the full unfoldment of our inner being. Any other type of Self-realization or empowerment is likely to be that of the ego, the mind or the time bound personality which keeps us limited to the realm of duality and sorrow.

Classical Yoga is a universal tradition aimed at the highest

Self-realization. This is not merely the fulfillment of our human potential but the realization of the universal Being as our true nature beyond body and mind. This extraordinary spiritual aim goes far beyond our usual personal, intellectual or religious concerns and aspirations. Such a 'spiritual Self-realization' is the ultimate goal of all embodied life that releases the soul from its bondage to karma, time and limitation, death and suffering. It is the realization of the Godhead or the Absolute, as both one with our own deepest consciousness and as the very essence of all that is or all that ever could be.

Through the insights of the inner Yoga, we journey from the transient and finite aspects of our nature as body and mind, to the eternal and the infinite reality as unconditioned consciousness and unbounded energy. For such a radical change to occur, we must set aside our ordinary thought processes and our personal ego in favor of an awareness that is not circumscribed by the brain or by the mind. We must open up to the entire universe—from the smallest subatomic particle to the vastest expanse of space—as our true home and deeper being.

This inner movement of transcendence is the real purpose of the many practices of Yoga from asana to deep meditation. Yoga shows us how to energize the forces of body, breath, heart and mind to propel us to a higher level of existence beyond them, not simply to make us content at the ordinary human level at which we usually dwell. To really practice Yoga, we must embrace this inner Yoga and all that it entails, which is to see all beings within our Self and our Self within all beings as the *Upanishads*, the scriptures of the ancient Yoga, eloquently proclaim:

"He who sees the Self in all beings and all beings in the Self henceforth has no disturbance. In the Knower for whom the Self has become all beings, where can there be any delusion or any sorrow for he who sees only the Oneness."[2]

Classical Yoga and the Cosmic Powers

Classical Yoga recognizes that we live in a Conscious Universe, pervaded by divine energies, including magical powers that modern science has not yet recognized. This Conscious Universe is the Purusha, the Supreme Being of all and the goal of all Yoga practices. Behind the physical forces of the universe—which have their own secret wisdom and extraordinary intricacy—are subtler powers of energy and information that we are just beginning to access in the high tech era from electricity to radio waves and atomic power.

Behind these forces of energy and information reside yet deeper powers of cosmic intelligence, bliss, awareness and being, extending beyond time, space, all possible worlds and all appearances. The greater universe is a mystical wonder of divine delight and blissful creativity, extending to multiple dimensions and interconnections within and without. Yoga requires ascending the ladder of these worlds to the Unborn and Uncreate beyond all manifestation, the world before the world as it were. This is not an abstract journey but requires awakening the universal Self within us.

In yogic thought, these great powers of the Conscious Universe are defined as *Devatas* or 'Divine principles', a term that is often rendered into the English language as 'Gods and Goddesses' or as 'deities'. The Devatas reflect the Divine consciousness that pervades all aspects of nature and our own psyche. They are powers of universal light and energy as archetypes, beings and forces all in one. We can contact them as principles, personalities or presences either externally or internally.

The Devatas or Gods and Goddesses reflect the great forces of nature from the five elements of earth, water, fire, air and ether. These elements form the root powers of creation up to the universal principles of time, space and energy according to the spiritual intelligence behind them. These deities endow the cosmic forces with faces and voices that can touch us personally and allow us to access their higher reality within our own consciousness. Yet beyond the manifest realm, the same deities reflect the various aspects of the Absolute; how the infinite and eternal Being-Consciousness-Bliss permeates the very fabric of existence and all that we can possibly experience.

Though the appearances of these deities in yogic texts—like the many forms of Shiva, the Goddess (Devi) or Vishnu—may seem alien or foreign to us in the West, they are not merely cultural forms or the icons of one particular religion opposed to another. The Devatas are symbolic expressions of the cosmic powers behind all life, which they mirror in diverse attributes, names and functions. They are the faces of Prana, the light of meditation, the beauty of bliss, the body of space, or the rhythms of peace, by way of a few poetic comparisons, not just the particular expressions of one community, belief system or another.

The symbolic appearances of these deities—which include naturalistic forms of animals, plants, rocks and stars as well as human forms with several arms, unusual ornaments and weapons—can seem bizarre to our modern minds. But it is meant to communicate to our inner being according to an intuitive language: the language of images, colors and gestures whose meaning is universal and beyond the definitions of any mere human dialect. Once we learn to grasp the cosmic relevance of symbolic representations, we can learn to work with them as easily as we can work with the outer forces of nature like wind or sunlight.

An inner communion with the deities is the basis of a real experiential Yoga practice, one that flows with deep energy and carries the blessings of all life. Yet besides the deities of the Yoga tradition—which are still full of life and energy—there are other deity traditions throughout the world, connected to greater or lesser degrees of energy and efficacy.

There are a number of Deity traditions in the West, starting with the pagan Gods and Goddesses in the older Greek, Roman, Celtic, Germanic and other native traditions of Pre-Christian Europe. Even the ancient Middle East, from which monotheistic traditions arose, contained many such traditions of deity worship that we see clearly in the iconography of ancient Egypt, Assyria, Babylonia or Sumeria. We can find deity worship in all indigenous and tribal religions—whether the Native American, African, Asian or Pacific Islanders—which occurs as part of their recognition of the sacred nature of all life.

We can discern similar light beings in the angels, saints and revelations of monotheistic traditions. We can find similar ethereal images in mystic poetry of all times and cultures. The Devatas are perhaps not as alien to our psyche as we might initially think but only to our current cultural mindset. Yet even in the modern media we look to stories of magic, myth and legend to entertain us, from ancient images to futuristic magic and science fiction. With a subtle shift of vision, each one of us can appreciate such Divine images and learn their secrets. This requires probing into the universal implications of their symbols, not just their outer forms, which ultimately rests upon the awakening of a deeper intuitive perception within us through contemplation and meditation.

Deity Yoga (Devata Yoga)

There is a simple key to approach the Gods and Goddesses and understand their deeper qualities: this is to recognize that there is but one power in the universe, which is a power of light and consciousness called *Shakti* in Sanskrit. The many deities are the receptacles of *Shakti*, the supreme energy of Consciousness, and represent its different forms and functions.

This Shakti is not only One in essence but unlimited in its manifestation, working on all levels of existence behind the forces of both nature and the psyche. The multiplicity of deities in the

Yoga tradition is an outcome of their representation of all aspects of Shakti—not only its underlying unity but its living rhythms, phases, interactions and intricacies.

The energies of the deities as ascending or descending, expanding or contracting, blissful or fierce, reflect specific states of consciousness or experiences that we must carefully traverse in our yogic quest, just as a seasoned mountain climber must cautiously move along the turns of his winding trail, though he is aware of the ultimate unity of his goal at the top of the peak. We cannot simply reduce these many deities to an abstract uniformity, though there is a greater Oneness behind them. The different powers that they hold must be honored in all their nuances.

The traditional name for the inner worship of the Devatas or Gods and Goddesses in the Yoga tradition is *Devata Yoga* or 'Deity Yoga', a practice that not only permeates the Hindu religion but which Tibetan Buddhists also employ and is central to all Tantric and Vedic traditions.

Deity Yoga involves working with the Divine powers outwardly through the forms and procedures of temple worship and inwardly through Yoga practices of pranayama, mantra and meditation. Through these processes, the Deities unfold the entire play of cosmic creation as well as revealing the path beyond the manifest world to the Absolute.

Many powerful temples in India still reverberate with the worship of their primary Devatas in elaborate rituals tied to the sacred Hindu calendar of festivals and holy days. Most Hindus in their homes worship the Gods and Goddesses in private shrines as well. Great Yogis honor the same deities within their own hearts as the Divine presence and power behind all.

Our own spiritual and yogic growth is the unfoldment of the deity, the God or Goddess within. Yoga is not about the development or glorification of our human personality and time bound ego, but that of the eternal soul potentials within us. To look to the Devata or inner Deity is perhaps the best way to open up to the flow of Divine grace. Through the Devata—the inner God and Goddess—we gain access to our true Self, which is one with all worlds, all creatures, all people and all the Gods.

Energies and Deities

As we begin to meditate deeply, we inevitably come into contact with the subtle forces of the deeper mind and heart. At first these powers may appear as forms of light or currents of energy imping-ing into our awareness in various flashes, vibrations and flows. This is our initial encounter with Shakti, which is the energy of awareness streaming down from the higher planes.

These spiritual energies often take the forms of Deities—Gods and Goddesses—in the imagistic and symbolic language of the universal mind. The Supreme Shakti, the background ruling pow-er itself, characteristically assumes the form of the Goddess as it has a feminine quality of beauty, charm and creativity: the Mother and Queen of all the worlds.

Because such deities reflect the Infinite and the Eternal be-yond the human sphere, they can appear frightening to our ordinary human mentality, whose preconceptions they transcend. Or they can appear supremely beautiful and blissful, a joy of an-other dimension than the body, mind and senses, which makes all worldly enjoyments seem meaningless.

While we may begin our spiritual journey with a philosophical idea of the Absolute or with an emotional faith in God or guru, as the real experiential path unfolds, it becomes a play of light, fire, and transformation. It is something more energetic than mental or emotional, a transformational encounter with a compelling power that causes us to go beyond ourselves and our idea of the world.

These inner forces can take human forms as great teachers and avatars, or as humanlike Gods and Goddesses. They can assume animal forms like the sacred bull, eagle, horse or serpent. They may appear as a combination of an animal head and a human body like the Hindu deity Ganesha with the head of an elephant. Or they may appear as an animal body with a human head like the great Sphinx of Egypt. They may take plant forms like the sacred cosmic tree whose roots are above in the eternal and whose branches are below in the world of time. Sometimes they take rock or mineral forms like mountains, caves or gems, or as the pillars, standing stones and obelisks of many ancient traditions.

As forms of the light, these spiritual powers can reflect the Sun, Moon, planets, stars or even just a common household fire. Going beyond representational forms, they can appear as mathematical patterns, geometrical designs, yantras, mandalas, flowers, or lotuses. Often these various dimensions are mixed together in a many-sided inner experience of a body streaming through space, a face appearing in the Sun, the voice of fire, the eye of lightning, or many others.

All these different Divine forms have a place in an inner Yoga practice. Yoga brings us in contact with them in various ways in its diverse methods and stages. Once we have entered into the stream of inner experience, their meanings will unfold and provide greater grace and guidance for us from within.

This has been my own experience as well. I originally approached Yoga from the profound philosophy of Vedanta, looking for the Absolute Brahman beyond all forms, which has remained the underlying foundation for all that I do. Yet as my practice of meditation developed, I came into contact with various forms of energy and light, which by degrees took on the appearance of different deities, notably the Goddess and Shiva.

Over years of practice, I came to experience the Goddess in her many forms, from the fierceness of Kali to the beauty of Sundari, not just as personifications of the feminine principle but as the inner powers of the world of nature, and the Shaktis of Brahman, the Absolute beyond. At the same time, I came in contact with Lord Shiva as the complimentary cosmic masculine force and universal will, as the very essence of light and life, and ultimately as the Being of all, the Absolute Brahman.

Once I had these inner experiences, all division between the Divine as form or formless or as personal or impersonal, broke down. The sense of myself as being separate from either nature or from the Absolute gradually dissolved. All boundaries of mere human identity faded into a greater universal Existence, leaving any attachments to the time and place far behind. I realized that the face of consciousness is present in all that we see and all that we can envision! The inner Yoga began to unfold according its own impetus as an ever-increasing current of Shakti and awareness, with its own voice, teaching and direction. Yoga practice became the dance of the inner Shakti moment by moment in the presence of the eternal Self of Shiva.

The Yoga of the Ishta Devata or Chosen Deity

So far we have discussed the Devata or inner deity in a general sense. Yet just as each human being has a unique form, personality and expression, so each Devata has its individuality and the different ways in which its energies unfold. Just as we can learn to understand the different personalities and talents of each person, so we can come to comprehend the special qualities of each deity.

The Gods and Goddesses come alive for those who work with them, who come to know them in an intimate and direct manner as living forces that enter into our daily experience and touch the very fabric of our existence. Each Devata has its own way of knowledge, its special appearance, gifts and powers and its special interaction with each individual.

Generally, a person chooses one primary Devata as the chief focus of his or her inner worship and practice. One particular Devata becomes our *Ishta*—our chief or chosen form of the Divine, our own special inner deity, for worship—to whom we give special attention. This *Ishta Devata* or personal deity assumes great importance relative to the spiritual path, providing the inner grace and assurance to help us proceed. *Devata or Deity Yoga is usually the Yoga of the Ishta Devata.* One could compare the role of the Ishta Devata with one's personal angel in western religions, but it is usually more intimate, a personal formation of divinity itself connected to our higher Self.

The great Yoga guru Patanjali states in the *Yoga Sutras*, the main classical textbook of Yoga, that the 'vision of the Ishta Devata' results from the practice of *Svadhyaya* or 'self-study'.[3] In this regard, Svadhyaya does not mean only self-study in the general sense, as it is usually translated but, rather, following the practices that are specific to our unique individual nature and temperament.[4] The vision of the Ishta Devata arises from studying the Divinity inherent within us, our own inner God or Goddess that is our deeper nature.

Patanjali also emphasizes *Ishvara Pranidhana* or 'surrender to the Divine within us' as a key component to Yoga practice and samadhi, which he refers to several times in the *Yoga Sutras*.[5] The worship of the Ishta Devata is an important means of connecting to Ishvara, who is not just God in an abstract or impersonal sense, but assumes specific forms in order to teach and guide us. The Ishta is our personal connection to Ishvara. The *Yoga Sutras* state that the fruit of Ishvara Pranidhana is samadhi, the Yogic state of absorption and realization that is the ultimate goal of practice.[6] The Ishta Devata is the best means to approach Ishvara and a key to the development of samadhi.

This means that the 'Yoga of the Ishta Devata' is an integral part of Classical Raja Yoga, though few Yoga teachers in the West teach it today, and many do not even know about it.

The Yoga tradition provides many Ishtas or personal deities to choose from, starting with the five main Hindu Devatas of Shiva, Vishnu, Devi (Goddess), Ganesha, and Surya (the Sun). Sometimes Buddha is added as the sixth. Rama and Krishna, along with the other avatars, come under Vishnu, while planetary deities come under Surya. The different forms of the Goddess like Kali, Durga, Lakshmi and Sarasvati come under the Devi. Shiva has many forms from the youthful Dakshinamurti to Yogeshvara as the Lord of Yoga to Nataraja as the cosmic dancer. Sometimes Skanda, the son of Shiva, represents another line. Sometimes Vedic deities like Indra, Agni and Soma form yet another.

However, any Divine power, principle, or representation from any enlightenment tradition, can become an Ishta Devata or personal form of the deity. Generally, Ishtas are formulations of the Divine in terms of a personal relationship as father or mother, brother, sister, friend, beloved, guru or master. The forms they assume usually develop out of these relationships.

The Ishta Devata should reflect our own inclinations, temperament, tendencies and manner of expression. *Ishta* means 'our choice' and so the Ishta cannot be imposed upon us by another, a group or an institution. In this regard, the Ishta is a very democratic phenomenon. We should be free to worship the Divine in whatever form we like, just as we should be free to live where we like, have the job that we like or vote for whomever we prefer. There is not just one Ishta Devata or personal deity for all, any more than there is just one food item or type of clothing for all.

This does not mean that we cannot follow the Divine form or manifestation honored by our family, guru or tradition as our own Ishta but, if we do so, it should be mirrored in our own hearts, not just done to please others. The Ishta or personal form of the deity is not a matter of external influences or trying to please others, but of our own Divine impulse regardless of what others may think. It is like choosing one's marriage partner. We should first examine the different Devatas carefully, perhaps working with several, before we decide upon one in particular as our Ishta. This choice should reflect the real wishes and deepest love of our inner being.

Once we have an inner connection to the Ishta, we are firmly planted on the yogic path and have a direct conduit to Divine grace and guidance. Once the Yoga is practiced in harmony with the inner deity, then the Yoga attains maturity, and assumes its own form, voice and expression. The Ishta Devata provides a steady flow of grace to guide our spiritual practice. It forms a link both to the Divine within and to the power of nature around us.

Personally, I follow the Goddess as my Ishta Devata as Kali, Durga and Sundari, in various forms in nature and as cosmic powers, not just as a human image. This was not so much the result of a personal choice, but of a continuous intuition of her presence and power from childhood, including several appearances of her before me. Connected to her was always Lord Shiva, who has a similar spectrum of manifestations from the anthropomorphic to the naturalistic and the abstract as a personification of Pure Being. Shiva has also come into my life in many ways, as the inner guide beyond the human realm and even beyond all form. Discovering Shiva and the Devi was not assuming a foreign religious identity for me but coming back to my true Self.

In following a particular Ishta Devata, one need not abandon all other Divine forms or spiritual approaches. One energizes the primary deity as a point of focus and integration for all other powers and practices. One learns to see the Ishta or chosen deity in all deities, extending to the Absolute beyond all manifestation.

The Devatas—the great Gods and Goddesses of the Cosmic Mind—look over this world and the karmas of the creatures that take birth within it. They constitute our spiritual family as manifestations of the Divine Father and Mother, the cosmic masculine and feminine forces who are our inner parents and prototypes. Working with them is helpful for all aspects of life, even ordinary goals like physical and psychological health and happiness.

Guru, Inner Deity and Self

Our examination has emphasized the Devata or inner deity as the basis of deeper Yoga practices, the awakening of cosmic energy within our deeper minds and hearts. However, most Yoga teachings today do not afford such significance to the deity. Some may not mention it at all.

Traditional Yoga practice rests upon three primary factors: the guru (spiritual teacher), the Devata (inner divinity) and the Self (Atman). All three are important, if not essential, though different yogic paths may emphasize one more than the others.

- The guru is the enlightened human teacher who provides instruction for the student and direction along the path.
- The Devata is the inner Divinity that we relate to—often conceived in a personal form—who provides the grace for our practice and guides us from within, our connection to God or Ishvara within us.
- The Self or Brahman is the ultimate goal or state of pure consciousness to be realized, who is the witness of all that we do.

These three factors are related: the guru's role is to guide the student both in communion with the inner deity and in the realization of the higher Self. The role of the Devata is to unfold the Divine powers within us leading us to the Self.

Of these three, the Devata is the least understood, though it is the most emphasized in ancient teachings. The guru provides the teaching and the Self is the goal but the Devata, one could say, is the path. The path proceeds largely through the inner deity, according to whom the internal awakening of energy or Shakti proceeds. The guru is the beginning of sadhana and the Self is the end, but the Devata works as the bridge between the two. The Devata mediates between the Guru and the Self and unites them together.

At a deeper level, one could say that there is only the Devata, the inner God or Goddess. The Devata is the inner Guru or spiritual power working within us. The outer guru is a reflection of this inner divinity in the external world. We need to awaken the Deity within us in order to perform the spiritual practice to reach to the higher Self that is the supreme divinity. Both guru and the disciple merge into the Devata which takes us to the *Atman*, our inner being of pure consciousness that is one with the Absolute.

Guru, Devata and Atman are aspects of the Devata as the Divine principle. The guru is the first Devata or divinity and the Self is the last or the supreme Devata. One moves from the 'Guru Devata', to the 'Ishta Devata' (inner Divinity), to the 'Atma Devata'. A true guru awakens the Devata within us and connects us to our own Ishta Devata as well as to the Divinity of our own Self.

We should not overlook the Devata in approaching the guru or the higher Self. It is the Devata that one should see in the guru, not just the human personality. Similarly, it is the Divine Self or Self as Devata (Atma Devata) that one is seeking, not merely the human or psychological Self. Unless one knows the Devata, one is likely to look at the guru and the Atman only in a personal sense. If one knows the Devata, then the guru is a channel of Divine grace and the Self is the supreme Divinity of the entire universe.

The Yoga of the Ishta Devata

The Devata is the real 'subject' of sadhana or spiritual practice. It is not the ego of the human being that can perform the sadhana aimed at eliminating the ego and letting the Inner Self shine forth. For Yoga sadhana, we need an inner power, a conduit to the Divine and our inner Self, in order to move the practice along. This is the place of the Devata. The path is the development of the Devata, its wisdom, power and grace as it moves us from our outer ego and self-image to the pure consciousness within us, beyond body and mind.

However, the Devata is also the real 'object or aim' of inner Yoga practice. The formless Self or Brahman cannot be the goal in any practical way because it is beyond time and space, cause and effect. The Devata as a power of the Self, however, can function as a recognizable goal. It has a form, energies and attributes that one can focus on stage by stage.

For those pursuing *Bhakti Yoga* or 'Yoga of devotion', the Devata as the chosen Divine form for worship is usually central. One worships the Goddess, Shiva, Krishna and so on as the primary focus of the mind and heart. Yet those following *Jnana Yoga* or the 'Yoga of Knowledge', which is formless in nature, can benefit from learning to work with the Devatas as representing cosmic and psychological principles, like the Dakshinamurti form of Shiva, who is said to be the guru of all the great sages.

For those practicing yogic methods of mantra, pranayama and meditation—the paths of Tantra and Kundalini Yoga—the Devata is equally central and serves to direct the inner flow of energy. *Kundalini Shakti*—the inner power of consciousness which such Yoga practices seek to arouse—is not just some internal electricity for the practitioner to personally manipulate; it is the presence and power of the Goddess within us, a sacred reality or Devata. Kundalini is the Divine Shakti which is the power of Yoga. The Yoga practitioner must learn to work with and surrender to the Shakti as the Goddess. Without understanding and connecting to Kundalini as a manifestation of the Goddess, one can run into many difficulties and not get beyond human desires and ambitions.

We live in a universe permeated by powerful forces of intelligence, with extraordinary Deities everywhere, whether it is in the clouds, the sands or in the distant nebulae. Connecting our hearts to them, the entire world will come alive as a play of Divine delight!

If we awaken the inner divinity, the God and Goddess within us, and bring back the Devata that modern Yoga has tended to neglect, our practice will gain a much higher meaning and efficacy. We are Shiva and the Goddess. We should not forget this. All formulations of divinity ever made by any person and culture are just aspects of our own deeper Self!

Let us not forget the Devatas, the great Gods and Goddesses and all formulations of Divinity, along our spiritual path! Let us learn to relate to the Divine within us with the same freedom and individualized approach that we are seeking in the rest of our lives! Let us learn to commune with the great powers of the Conscious Universe, allowing the forces of nature speak to us and lead us back through the heart of creation to the Supreme Reality!

The Gods and Goddesses as Forms of Brahman

Hindu Gods and Goddesses—with their magical appearances and superhuman powers—are usually treated by modern scholars in a superficial manner as personifications of the forces of nature, or merely as imaginary spirits invented by the unscientific mind. Other deity traditions in the world are denigrated in the much same manner from ancient Egypt to the Native American, which are similarly designated as primitive.

Present day academics prefer to examine these deities according to the concerns of modern psychology or anthropology in which any cosmic and yogic meaning is lost. These indirect interpretations of such scholars should not be confused with the views of practitioners who work with these Divine energies in an experiential manner, which is what we will explore here.

Hindu Gods and Goddesses represent the great cosmic powers, the inner Divine energies inherent throughout the universe. They are part of the Yoga of the Ishta Devata or the inner God and Goddess. These deities are not separate Gods but forms or manifestations of God, Ishvara, the Cosmic Lord and Creator. They represent the various powers and qualities of the Divine, or different ways of relating to it. They are the principles of *Bhakti Yoga*, the Yoga of Devotion. The wealth of different Devatas represents the richness of the Hindu path of devotion that allows us to access the Divine in all possible forms and manners, rejecting nothing that links us together with the higher forces.

Yet besides indicating aspects of the Cosmic Lord, Hindu Gods and Goddesses are aspects of Brahman, the impersonal Godhead beyond the manifest universe. In this regard, the Devatas are powers of *Jnana Yoga*, the Yoga of Knowledge. They portray how that supreme reality of Pure Existence can be contacted through the forces of nature, both in the outer world and in our own minds and bodies.

One may ask: *How can Gods and Goddesses, which are usually formulated as personalities, be a manifestation of an Impersonal Being, Power and Existence?* If we look deeply, we can discern that their forms and personalities are but symbols of something beyond form and personality. This is why their forms and personalities are extraordinary, supernatural and multifaceted, often magical or even terrible in their appearances.

Vedic Devatas and Brahman

The Vedic tradition is the older tradition in India and later traditions, including Yoga, Vedanta and Tantra, reflect various aspects of Vedic knowledge and practice, particularly Vedic rituals and mantras. Vedic Deities are primarily powers of light. The four main Vedic Devatas in their light forms are *Agni* (Fire), *Vayu* or *Indra* (Lightning or Wind), *Surya* (Sun) and *Soma* (Moon). These light forms possess broad correspondences in the universe as a whole, as the powers of matter, life, mind and consciousness. They do not simply indicate outer forms in the natural world.

Agni stands for transformative heat on all levels from the fire on Earth to the digestive fire in creatures, to the fire of consciousness itself (Chidagni). Vayu indicates all vibratory movement from the wind in the atmosphere to the Prana in living beings, to the energy currents in cosmic space, to the very breath of pure existence, Brahman. Surya indicates the supreme principle of light, whether the Sun in the sky, the eye in the body, or the perceptive power of the higher Self. Soma is the reflective aspect of light from the Moon in the sky, to the contemplative power of the mind, to bliss itself, Ananda.

Brahman, the supreme Godhead in the *Upanishads*, is compared to a great fire, from which all worlds and creatures arise as but sparks. "That is the truth, just as from a well-burning fire, similar sparks come forth a thousandfold; so too, from the Eternal various beings arise and to in it return."[7]

Brahman is also compared to the Wind or Vayu, a formless force that when it blows creates and moves everything in existence. "Reverence to Vayu, you are the manifest form of Brahman."[8] Brahman is said to be like the Sun, the supreme source of light, life and consciousness. The *Upanishads* say, "Worship the Sun as Brahman."[9] Such correlations do not mean that Brahman is limited to the powers of the natural world, but rather that such cosmic powers are manifestations of Brahman, symbols of the supreme light that we can follow out in order to discover its transcendent nature. In this regard, the *Upanishads* also state, "The Being (Purusha) in the Sun, he am I."[10]

If we look deeply into the inner reality of the Vedic deities, they lead us to Brahman as the supreme light of existence. Agni or Fire is *Brahmagni*, the inextinguishable immortal fire of Brahman and the undying light of pure existence.[11] Vayu is the formless being, space and power of Brahman. Surya or the Sun is Brahman as the light that illumines all, the Sun that neither rises nor sets but dwells forever in an eternal day of spiritual light. Soma is Brahman as pure delight, unlimited calm and contentment.

These forces reveal the Absolute in the language of light just as later Vedantic and Buddhist philosophies used logic and abstract terminology. But we must understand their symbolism in order to appreciate this. Yet, perhaps more importantly, these powers of light are indicative of the inner energies of Yoga and Tantra. The Sun, Moon, Fire and Lightning are inner energy centers of the heart, head, root chakra and third eye, as we will discuss later in the book.

Hindu and Yogic Theism

The deities of classical Hindu thought[12] are articulated in a theistic fashion, emphasizing God or the Cosmic Lord, Ishvara as the Supreme Being working behind the universe and its laws.[13] Ishvara is the Creator, Preserver and Destroyer of the entire universe, as well as the original guru of the yogic path according to the *Yoga Sutras*.[14] He is the Divine guide that we can commune with and become one with in our own hearts.

However, between Hindu theism and western religious theism, at least in its dominant forms, are two main differences. First, Ishvara works through the law of karma and rebirth, and does not just afford one life to the soul. Second, Ishvara has many names, forms and functions and can be addressed as male or female, and appears through many great avatars and sages. The One God of the *Vedas* is not opposed to the many Gods and Goddesses, which are but its different manifestation on various levels and with different qualities.

Yet Hindu thought does not end with theism, however exalted that may be. The cosmic creator or God with qualities (Saguna Brahman) is a manifestation of the formless Brahman, the Godhead beyond creation, or God without qualities (Nirguna Brahman). The manifest universe is but waves at the surface of the greater reality of Brahman which itself never undergoes any change. In the Supreme Brahman, all becomes one, including God, the soul and the world.

Our own soul or inner Self also has these two same aspects as with or without qualities. The individual soul (Jivatman) or reincarnating entity is connected to the Creator or Ishvara and consists of a portion of its energy. It takes birth to help work out the Divine will in creation. But our deepest Self is beyond all birth and death and is one with the supreme Self (Paramatman) and with Brahman, the unborn Absolute.

These two aspects of Self and Divinity as with or without qualities are connected. Traditional Yoga aims at the realization of the supreme Self or Brahman as its highest goal. But it proceeds through the help, grace and guidance of Ishvara or God, particularly in the form of various Ishta Devatas or Gods and Goddesses.

Ishvara has three primary forms or manifestations at a cosmic level according to the great Hindu trinity of the *Brahma*, the Creator, *Vishnu*, the Preserver, and *Shiva*, the Destroyer or Transformer. These are not three separate Gods, but the three aspects of Ishvara, relative to the gunas or prime qualities of Rajas (creation-expression), Sattva (maintenance-protection) and Tamas (destruction-transformation). Of these three aspects of Ishvara, it is Shiva that is the closest to the supreme Brahman or the Absolute because he is closest to the formless state.

Shiva and Kali as the Formless Brahman

We can examine the Hindu trinity from another angle. Shiva is 'Nirguna Brahman' or pure existence beyond all qualities. Vishnu is 'Ishvara', God as the Cosmic Lord or 'Saguna Brahman'. Brahma as 'Mahat Tattva' or Cosmic Mind out of which creation springs and which is the basis of cosmic law or Dharma. Shiva himself is called *Maheshvara*, the great Ishvara, and *Parameshvara*, the supreme or higher Ishvara, which further connects him with Brahman.

Shiva as a deity, one could say, is the personification of the supreme Brahman, the impersonal formless Absolute reflected in a personal form and symbolism. At a higher level, Shiva represents transcendent pure consciousness, pure existence, and immutable peace—inherently beyond and not connected with anything in the realm of time and space, birth and death. He is beyond all the dualities, including good and evil, and is present in suffering as well as all joy.

As Shiva is beyond all conceptions, he is often portrayed in an unpredictable and paradoxical manner. He is a great ascetic, yet is also the higher God of love. He is the God of healing, but can also cause great pain. He is the bringer of peace, but also casts the most terrible arrow. He has the purest light but does not shrink from the darkness. He brings us our highest good, yet does not bow down to any simplistic moral code of good and evil. He works to take us beyond any boundaries that we would put upon him or upon ourselves. He demands that we surrender our limited mind and ego to the Absolute.

In the same way as the trinity of great Gods, Hindu thought recognizes the primacy of three great Goddesses connected to them, the Goddess *Sarasvati* of Brahma or the Creator, Goddess *Lakshmi* of Vishnu or the Preserver, and Goddess *Kali* for Shiva as the Destroyer-Transformer. Of these three, Shiva's wife Kali, like Shiva himself, is the closest to the formless Brahman and can similarly function as its personification.

Kali is Brahman's supreme Shakti beyond all barriers, divisions and constraints. She represents the pure power of existence, which as the infinite and eternal, permeates all space and time and yet dwells beyond it. Kali's terrible appearance signifies her transcendent nature that breaks down all the transient enjoyments that we are attached to. Her garland of skulls shows her ruling over suffering and death and her ability to take us beyond them. The head chopper that she carries as a weapon is adorned with an eye, indicating that it is the power of spiritual insight to cut through all negativity and duality.

Kali represents the calming and silencing of the mind that is the essence of the inner Yoga. She symbolizes the highest state of *nirodha* or mergence in the *Yoga Sutras*,[15] *nirvana* or dissolution in Buddhism, and *Brahma-nirvana* or dissolution in Brahman of the

Bhagavad Gita.[16] She indicates the prana or life-force merged into itself, the ending of death in the ending of birth! Kali is the very breath of Brahman that occurs without breathing, sustaining everything silently within itself. She is not simply the force of nature or Prakriti and her three gunas but the pervasive power of the Supreme beyond all change and fluctuation.

Because of their connections with the Supreme Brahman, Shiva and Kali are not clearly defined personalities but personifications of higher principles and powers. They do not act in a normal way or take on ordinary appearances. They can appear in forms that appear harsh or terrible to us, with weapons, blood or wrath. Shiva and Kali represent the impersonal in its first manifestation towards personality. They break down the personality into the infinite. This is why their forms do not conform to any rules, order or stereotyped patterns. They embody the transcendent which, from the standpoint of the manifest or phenomenal world, must be paradoxical, cataclysmic and transformational in its effects.

Shiva and Kali take us beyond Sattva guna or pure and virtuous conduct to pure existence or *Sat* beyond all actions. To do this they must violate or show the limitations of the outer cosmic order. Even the beautiful personal forms of the Divine are limitations that we must go beyond in order to reach the Supreme. Shiva and Kali will break down our attachment to these forms in order to move our awareness beyond all dualities. Shiva and Kali take us back to Brahman in which they merge together. They represent light and energy as the most primal forces, the peace and power of the infinite in which all universes are but passing waves.

Deity Yoga as the Yoga of Brahman

To really see the Devatas (Gods and Goddesses) is to perceive them as forms of Brahman. Each Deity is a doorway to the infinite which is Brahman. Each indicates a path beyond form and personality through reflecting a primal or archetypal form, power or personality.

Generally, the 'Yoga of Brahman' is an approach of *Jnana Yoga* or the 'Yoga of Knowledge', which proceeds mainly through meditation on pure Being. But Devata Yoga can also be a part of the Yoga of Brahman. This occurs when we see the Devata (deity) as a symbolic and energetic formation of Brahman (the Absolute). The Devatas work to take us to Brahman by expanding our personality into the impersonal. They do this through their personifications of cosmic powers that expand our human personality into the impersonal Absolute. The Devatas are the prime forces at work on all levels of existence in order to lead us to that Being which is everywhere. They are the many sides of Brahman in manifestation.

Brahman is the essence of all our faculties. It is the "ear of the ear, the mind of the mind, the speech of speech, the breath of the breath, and the eye of the eye," as the *Upanishads* say.[17] It is heat in fire, the wetness in water, the movement in air, and the stability of the earth. The Devatas also represent such essences of cosmic action and experience. When we perceive their essences, rather than just their outer forms, we see Brahman.

In the Supreme Brahman, all the prime factors of existence—the Self, the Devata, God, the Guru and the world—merge into Unity. The waves fall into the sea. The different rays return to the one light of the Sun. Brahman is present as the Being in everything from the smallest particle of dust to the brightest star. Touching that pure Being, each thing in the universe becomes a Devata or deity for us and we can connect ourselves with Divine currents working in the forces of nature, light, time, space and all the yearnings of the human heart. The Many become the One and the One smiles through all diversity without any change of its infinite immutable nature.

When we look at the Gods and Goddesses, we should always remember the presence of pure light and pure being, the infinite Brahman behind them. The Devatas are doorways into this infinite unknown and unborn, which we should traverse through with grace.

Learn to see the formless behind the form, the nameless behind the name, the impersonal behind the personality, Brahman behind the Devata. Then the Absolute and the relative world will merge together in your awareness into a magical vision of endless delight!

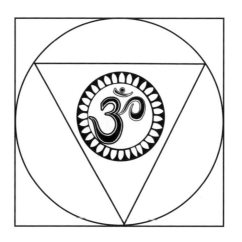

Atma Devata: The Self as the Supreme Divinity

The sense of self is not something unique to our species. It is common to all living creatures, each of which seeks to express and to perpetuate itself. Beyond embodied life, the sense of self pervades the entire universe as the very ground of Being, which is Self-existence. The sense of self is the root of our minds, emotions and prana. The inner Yoga aims at helping us realize the higher Self hidden within us, so that we can move from our human ego to the cosmic presence as our real identity.

In the modern world, psychology dominates our thinking and shapes how we view spirituality. We have come to look upon the Atman or higher Self in a psychological light as a formation of human emotions, not as a cosmic reality. Psychology is mainly concerned with the ego-self and bringing it to a state of harmony and happiness. Yoga, however, is aimed at going beyond the ego-self to the Self that is unconditioned, beyond body and mind, and transcends birth and death.

True spirituality is the quest for our true nature in pure consciousness, which is real Self-knowledge and Self-realization, not simply about achieving balance within the field of the personal self and its social urges. True Self-knowledge is something much more than any psychological knowledge; it is a universal and cosmic awareness, not just a knowledge of emotion, sexuality or our personal traumas.

Today many groups are working to psychologize spirituality; to make it into a subtle form of psychological therapy, analyzing anger, fear and desire as the prime factors of the inner quest. On the positive side, this encounter between psychology and spirituality can help to spiritualize psychology, bringing Yoga and meditation into psychological approaches for treating emotional disturbances, neuroses and traumas. Indeed, Yoga and its related system of Ayurvedic medicine can add many practical methods and deeper insights on how to deal with psychological problems, greatly expanding our variety of treatments and allowing the patient a greater role in healing themselves.[18]

Yet on the negative side, a psychological approach can confuse yogic spirituality with mere human emotional urges. It can reduce our spiritual Self or soul to the confines and concerns of the ego and our outer nature as a social or political entity. At the worst, it reduces yogic spirituality to a human psychological problem, as if higher yogic states of awareness were some psychological disturbance or cult.

Our true Self is not the psychological self or ego that is to be discarded for it to shine forth. Our true Self is not the personal identity of this particular incarnation. It is not the self-formation of emotion or the product of our personal likes and dislikes. It is not our mental or intellectual identity through the opinions, beliefs and predilections of our thought processes. It is not even our human self but our eternal soul that unites us to all beings and all worlds.

The Self as the God or Goddess Within Us

To put it simply: *our true Self or Atman is a Devata or Divine principle.* The Self is a principle of sentience, awareness and self-being inherent in all existence. It is the ultimate principle behind all the laws, principles and dharmas operative in this magical universe of mind, energy and matter.

Our true Self is a divinity, a God or Goddess, the Divine power behind all time, space and causation. We are God. God is our true nature. We are Divine beings with all the powers of the universe within us. Yet this Divinity is not a theological principle or religious belief but the very nature of existence that is self-aware, self-determining and self-responsible. This Atman or Self is Brahman, the Absolute Being-Consciousness-Bliss.

An important yogic approach common to both Veda and Tantra is to approach our true Self as a Divinity. This is to honor the Divine presence within yourself—to respect your own being and consciousness as sacred, immortal and untainted. It is to contact the God or Goddess within you and seek to align your awareness, motivation and behavior according to its wisdom and grace. You are Shiva and Shakti and can find their grace by being true to your highest aspirations and deepest wishes!

From Psychology to Yogic Spirituality

From the standpoint of psychology, worship of the inner Self can be an adulation of the ego, ignoring our personal faults and abrogating our social responsibilities. It is little more than a fantasy to cover over facing the hard realities of our emotional nature. Yet such psychological reductionism can also be rigid and can cut off the roots of spiritual aspiration and idealism within us. It can make us dry, lacking in devotion, and unable to project any higher vision beyond the neurotic mind.

The real problem is not our true Self and individuality but the false self that consists of our identification with the external world and its transient conditions. The Self is the source of light and life, love and wisdom within us. The ego is the externalized self born of desire that causes us to seek happiness on the outside and lose our inner peace.

We do not need to give up our true Self, which is the Divinity within us, in order to find truth and happiness. We need only remove the wrong notion of who we are, which is the limiting of our true self to a particular creaturely identity. Be your Self. Be true to your Self. But make certain that it is the inner Self, not the outer self-promoting, self-glorifying ego!

An important law of the mind is that whatever we focus our attention on that we tend to become. Whatever we give our greatest attention to in life is, one could say, is the Divinity we aspire to become. The danger in fixating on the neurotic psychological self is that we may end up reinforcing it; we can get lost in its peculiarities, traumas and idiosyncrasies. We can give more power to the psychological self rather than dissolving it.

We should worship the true Self within us as the Self of all beings, as the Being behind all existence and the light of all the worlds. This vision can take us in an instant beyond our human problems, however insoluble or intractable these may appear. Our problems are inherent in our psychology which focuses on our personal identity as our true reality, dividing us from God, nature and each other. We cannot get beyond these problems without opening up to that in us which inherently transcends them.

We must learn to set the psychological self aside, which is also to see the universal forces, the elements and qualities at work within our bodies and minds, not simply to take our personal history or education as who we really are. All of nature works within us according to a secret intelligence. Even our psychological self is an aspect of nature's energy and expression, elements and gunas, not something that belongs uniquely to us.

Our psychological self has its place as a vehicle of expression and action for the soul in the physical world. But focusing on the psychological self as our true nature will no more take us to the eternal truth than will focusing on our physical bodies. We can grant the psychological self its appropriate place in our outer lives as a mechanism of personal existence but should not confuse it with our true reality which is beyond time, space and person.

Feel free to let your personal self aside and become one with all! Feel free to give up your likes and dislikes, joys and sorrows and find contentment in your own inner being beyond all gain and loss. Be selfless in the true sense, which is to be true to the Divine Self within you and let the human ego fade away. Discover your greater Self in all of nature, in the plants, rocks, and animals, in the clouds, stars, galaxies and beyond.

Assert your true universal Self and let go of all false appearances, pretensions and efforts to please others. Let your self-sense naturally expand like the wind through the release of your breath to the most distant horizon. Unite the light of your mind and senses with the light of the sun and stars.

Your true Self is the pure light of awareness beyond body and mind. It gives light, life and love to all creatures and brings beauty and bliss to the entire universe. Accept that light within and cease dwelling in its shadows in your outer existence.

Worship the true Self within you. Just as you offer flowers or prayers to the Divinity of your choice, do so to the Self as the divinity within. See the Devata in your Self and your Self in the Devata. Let Shiva, Krishna, Devi, or whatever Divine form you worship, be reflected in your own nature.

Honor yourself. Respect your being. Acknowledge your integrity as an eternal soul. *Bring out the God and Goddess within you.* Live the Divine Life intended for you. Use the tools of Yoga to unfold the Devata, the inner Deity or Divine Presence within you that is the Self of the entire universe. Then the cosmic energy or Divine Shakti will flow within you in all its vitality, perception and bliss.

The Devatas or cosmic powers are more your real Self than is your psychological self. Learn to be one with that Atma Devata in all the Devatas. Let your true Self reflect all the Gods and Goddesses, Gurus and Avatars, which are its manifestations. Unfold your Divine being and beauty with fearlessness and delight.

Be yourself the God or Goddess that is your deepest reality and true dignity as a Divine expression. Do not forget your true Self in the worship of the Divine. Yet remember that all the powers of nature and divinity are but aspects of your own true nature, the Divine Sun of which your human life is but a single ray!

Shiva and Shakti: the Guiding Deities of the Inner Yoga

Yoga is a seeking of union with the Divine within. As such, there are inner Divine powers ruling over the practice of Yoga and facilitating its internal transformations. Shiva and Shakti—the Great God and Great Goddess, *Mahadeva* and *Mahadevi*—are personifications of these great powers of Yoga, which reflect the higher realities working behind and beyond all the forces of the universe.

Shiva and Shakti represent the Being and Energy of Pure Consciousness beyond time and space and how we can experience them as the two sides of our deepest nature. This is not to say that other deities cannot have such roles, but that these two can be specially understood in this manner. Working with the universal Shiva-Shakti energies is one of the main paths of Yoga in all of its aspects as knowledge, devotion or special Yoga techniques.

Shiva is *Yogeshvara*, the great Lord of Yoga. Shakti is the *Yoga Shakti* or power of Yoga. Using a Jungian approach, we could say that Shiva and Shakti are the archetypes of Yoga within us, the ideal Yogi and Yogini. By awakening Shiva and Shakti, the God and the Goddess, the Yogi and the Yogini within us, we can set in motion all the dynamic currents of inner growth and transformation, allowing their energies to spiral within us along their natural ascent into the Infinite.

Shiva and Shakti are reflected in the cosmic masculine and feminine forces in all creatures and so are intimately connected with sexuality. Yet beyond these biological forces, they represent the two primary forces in nature as the mountain and the valley, the Sun and the Moon, fire and water and all other such innumerable variations in this world of duality built upon complementary forces. Shiva and Shakti, like yin and yang, represent the prime duality behind all energies in the universe. To truly understand them requires much more than merely looking at them in human or sexual terms. It requires understanding the whole of reality, manifest and unmanifest, and all its diverse powers and principles.

Yet Shiva and Shakti are not just inert forces or abstract principles, they have a personal reality for us as the Divine Father and Divine Mother. This is probably the easiest way to understand them. Shiva and Shakti can appear to us in personal forms and we can commune with them as with another being. We can see them, talk to them, and feel their energy and love around us. Shiva and Shakti exist both as personal potentials within us and as cosmic powers outside us. We can approach them on both personal and impersonal levels, pervading all aspects of existence, animate and inanimate.

There is much yogic knowledge that comes to us in the form of teachings about Shiva and Shakti. One of the most important of these is that yogic power (Shakti) arises from inner peace (Shiva). Shiva symbolizes the silent meditative mind and Shakti indicates the powerful creative energy which flows from it. Shakti is the power of inner peace that becomes a channel for the cosmic powers of the greater universe of consciousness and bliss to flow into us.

True Shakti is not the power born of restlessness, aggression or conflict. She is the power born of concentration, devotion and compassion. In this regard, we should not confuse Shakti with outer forms of power based upon ego, self-assertion and violence. Shakti is the power that unifies and spiritualizes, not the power that divides or destroys. What Shakti does destroy is negativity, the forces of ignorance, duality and hatred. In the process, she upholds all that is creative, transformative and compassionate.

While we may primarily worship either Shiva or Shakti, we should always offer homage to both. Only when Shiva and Shakti come together does the real bliss flow. Apart from Shakti, the awareness of Shiva remains transcendent and cannot help us. Apart from Shiva, the power of Shakti has no support or receptacle to hold its energy within us.

Uniting Shiva and Shakti means uniting Shiva and Shakti within ourselves as the consciousness (Shiva) and power (Shakti) of Yoga, and as all aspects of the dualities of our nature from male and female, to fire and water, mind and emotion, activity and receptivity. One of the best ways to do this is to visualize the right half of our body as Shiva and the left half as Shakti as in the form of *Ardhanareshvara*, which means God who is half male and half female, the form of Shiva with Shakti as his left side.

There are many great teachings relative to Shiva and Shakti throughout the *Vedas, Upanishads, Puranas, Tantras* and yogic literature like the *Yoga Upanishads*. There are many ways to work with their forces through ritual, pilgrimage, mantra, pranayama, yantra and meditation. Nearly half the billion Hindus in the world are primarily worshippers of Shiva and Devi, complementing the others who are mainly devoted to Vishnu and Lakshmi.

Most importantly, once we establish a connection with Shiva and Devi as deities inside ourselves, they become our inner teachers and can guide us directly along our special path. We learn to perceive their workings in all of life and nature. Once this occurs, we transcend outer forms of practice and a spontaneous flow opens up that carries us along according to a higher law. We experience the deities as aspects of our own inner being and its expression through all that we do.

The deities add a richness to Yoga practice both in terms of knowledge and energy. And their powers are not far away or alien; they pervade all that we do as the forces of life. They are inherent in the movement of the inhalation and exhalation of the breath, in the interplay of reason and emotion in the mind, and in the ascent of the soul's aspiration and the descent of Divine grace. We need only sincerely to call on them and they will respond immediately!

Once we bring the energies of Shiva and Shakti into our Yoga, our practice will gain a new meaning, intensity and focus. The entire universe will be with us, and the great movements of eternal time and cosmic transformation will be mirrored in every moment that we experience as a manifestation of Divine wonder. May the supreme Shiva and the most blissful Shakti arise within you in their magical dance beyond all limitation!

The Shiva Linga and the Shakti Yoni: Symbols of the Two Primal Powers

Sexuality is the strongest of our biological and psychological forces. Yet it reflects greater and higher powers, the energies of cosmic consciousness of which it is only an outer manifestation. The polarity that we discover in sexuality is mirrored in the great dualities of nature from electricity and magnetism, to fire and water, to the sun and the moon, and such natural forms as the mountain and the valley.

Working with this universal polarity in order to reach the pure unity behind it is the basis of real Tantric Yoga. Sexuality is an important force that we must understand in the process, whether we choose to express it in a human relationship or renounce it for a solitary path. But sexuality is not the be all and end all of Tantric Yoga. *Real Tantric Yoga consists of unfolding the Divine powers within ourselves, the inner God and Goddess, whose natures are the light and energy of consciousness.*

The two main Tantric symbols are the *Shiva linga* and the *Shakti yoni*, which indicate the main ascending and descending forces in the universe. They have many forms on all levels of manifestation. Understanding them is central to the inner Tantric Yoga and its transformative processes. While the linga and the yoni on a biological level are symbols of sexual energy, male and female, this is only a portion of their greater symbolism as the two prime powers of cosmic existence. It is not all that they are, as some would think, or their main indication.

The Shiva linga is often portrayed in an upright conical form like the male sexual organ. Indeed, some Shiva lingas are quite phallic in their appearance and the linga is often called a phallic symbol by scholars. However, there are many other types of lingas which are circular, elliptical, triangular or columnar in form. The linga is the symbol of the Shiva principle of immutability, stability, strength and endurance, which is reflected in the cosmic masculine principle, the higher side of masculine values and virtues. The sexual side of the linga is not the essence of its meaning. And great devotees of the Shiva linga have their minds and hearts far beyond the type of phallic cults, which is all that some scholars see.

In the Sanskrit language, the word *linga* refers to a 'chief mark' or 'characteristic' of something. The term is nowhere simply a synonym for the male sexual organ. Linga indicates what is outstanding and determinative. In this regard, the male sexual organ can be said to be the distinguishing characteristic or linga of a man at a physical level, but many other such marks of distinction exist on various levels.

In Yoga philosophy, the term 'linga' refers to the subtle body, which is the dominant principle in our nature over the physical body, as it is the subtle body, not the physical body, which is re-born.[19] The Shiva linga can symbolize this subtle or light body, which has an egg like form. The linga can also indicate the upper spinal region from the heart to the head where the influence of the subtle body predominates. The linga is a place where energy is held, generated and sustained.

Similarly, the term 'yoni' in Sanskrit means a place of origin in general. *Brahma-yoni*, for example, is Brahman or the Absolute as the source of creation. The female sexual organ can be said to be the yoni or creative center of the woman. But the term yoni does not necessarily indicate the female sexual organ or primarily indicate that to those who use it as a sacred symbol. While on a biological level, the yoni is the womb, in its greater symbolism it is also a cave, a valley, a place of origins, and the matrix of space and time. To translate linga and yoni in purely sexual terms does not do justice to their Sanskrit meanings and brings about many needless distortions!

The problem is that the modern mind—particularly under the influence of Freudian psychology—uses sexuality as its primary means of interpreting life, but regarding it only as a physical force. It even looks at sexual behavior for understanding higher domains of life like art and spirituality, emphasizing sexual symbolisms or examining the sex life of the persons involved in these pursuits in order to explain their higher experiences! This 'sexual reduction-ism' misses the deeper sensitivities and inspirations of the soul within us. Clearly sexuality is there for everyone, but real spiritu-ality and genuine creativity are not so easy![20]

Symbolism of the Linga and the Yoni

The Shiva linga represents the ascending energy of consciousness and life in nature. We see this in such forms as the mountain, the thunder cloud, the tree, and the upright human being. Many lin-gas enshrined in Hindu temples like that at Kedarnath, the most important Shiva site in the Himalayas, are rocks in the shapes of small mountains. Other lingas are associated with light: the lingas of the Sun, Moon and Fire. There are twelve famous *Jyotir lingas* or 'light forms' of Shiva at twelve special temples throughout India.

The Tamil Nadu state in South India has special Shiva linga forms for the five elements with lingas of earth, water, fire, air and ether at special temples in the region. Arunachala, the sacred hill of Ramana Maharshi, is the fire linga of Shiva, of which Ramana was said to be a manifestation.

Yet other Shiva lingas are associated with gold or crystal, the light powers in the metal kingdom. The Shiva linga is often de-scribed in terms of light, crystal or transparency. Shiva himself is said to be pure light or light in its primal undifferentiated state,[21] from which the diversified lights of the Sun, Moon and Fire arise.

The Shiva linga is connected to the upward pointed triangle, which is also the symbol of fire. The linga is present in the male sexual organ both in plants and in animals. But we should not ignore its other forms. The worship of the linga is more generally a worship of pillars, obelisks, standing stones and pyramids. Tantric linga worship is connected to Vedic pillar worship,[22] which has parallels throughout the ancient world and in indigenous cultures in general, who can still perceive the spiritual powers behind the formations of nature.

The Shiva linga is often a pillar of light. In special Vedic fire rituals, the fire can be made to rise in the shape of a pillar which can take the shape of a man! In fact, the term Dharma originally refers to what upholds things and can be symbolized by a pillar. The Shiva linga is the universal pillar of Dharma or Dharma linga. The pillar is also an inner symbol indicating the erect spine and concentrated mind.

In terms of our human nature, there are several lingas or characteristic marks. The force of Prana is the linga or pillar force upholding the physical body, according to the currents that emanate from it. This is the inner *Prana Linga*. Our deeper intelligence or Buddhi provides us the power of insight to discern higher realities, the *Buddhi Linga*. The Atman or higher Self is the ultimate linga or determinative force of our nature that remains steady and elevated (transcendent) throughout all of our life experience, the *Atma Linga*.

The Shakti yoni is the complementary horizontal force to the Shiva linga's vertical force. The yoni is the valley to the mountain, the meadows to the forests, the water to the fire, the woman to the man. Geometrically, the yoni is the downward pointing triangle, which also indicates water, creation, the flow of grace, Soma or nectar. The yoni is present as the female sexual organ in both plants and animals as the power of the womb. The yoni of the Goddess is worshipped at the great temple of Kamakhya in the state of Assam in northeast India, where a special spring of water flows on a small hill by the great Brahmaputra River.

The worship of the yoni is part of the greater worship of sacred circles and ring stones which, along with standing stones, we find everywhere in the ancient world. Stonehenge in England, and other similar sacred sites that have standing stones formed into great circles, show the union of the linga and the yoni or the cosmic male and female principles. They reflect the universal religion of the two powers that the Hindus call Shiva and Shakti.

The real inner yoni is the cave or small space within the heart (dahara akasha) in which the entire universe dwells and which holds the deepest inner fire within us and the very well springs of life. To merge one's mind into that yoni of the heart is to move through all creation to the Absolute beyond, to be reborn into the Supreme!

The linga and the yoni always go together, first of all on the level of opposites. The linga with the yoni below it shows the union of male and female energies, not just in sexuality, but also as electro-magnetic forces, with the currents of circular Shakti entwining the still upright linga, like an electrical energy transformer. Each serves to support and sustain the other.

The linga in its movement creates a yoni, just as a point in its movement creates a circle. We can see this in the circular movement of the stars, planets and nebulae, as well as in many other diverse phenomena in the world of nature. The central luminary is the linga and its field of revolution is the yoni. The planets form a yoni or circle as they revolve around the Sun as the linga, of the solar system, its central principle or axis. Yet the Sun itself is revolving around other stars and creating a yoni or circle of its own.

Uniting the linga and the yoni is not just a matter of sexuality but of uniting the centrifugal force (linga) with the centripetal force (yoni), or uniting the electric force of Shiva with the magnetic (attractive) force of Shakti. It is uniting the center with the periphery, so that the One and the Infinite merge into a single experience.

The linga and the yoni are united in the chakra or the wheel, with the linga as the axis and the yoni as the circumference. The Hindu usage of chakras in ritual and in art also reflects the union of these two powers. Similarly, each chakra of the subtle body shows the union of the Shiva and Shakti energies operative at its particular level of manifestation. There are various other lingas and yonis in the chakras that hold the inner keys to yogic energies.

The spine itself is an inner Shiva linga through which currents of Shakti flow. Or, from another perspective, Shiva and Shakti are the two currents of energy through the spine, with the force Shiva following an upward and concentrating motion and the Shakti force a horizontal, circular and downward movement. Together they form the various lotuses of the chakras as a spiral of energies.

The Linga, the Yoni and the Yantra

The linga and the yoni are part of a greater mathematical symbolism that is embodied in the figure of the *yantra*, the geometrical meditation devices of Tantric Yoga. Each deity has its own yantra for worship, which represents its subtle body, as opposed to its visualized human form that represents its gross body. The yantra also indicates the energy pattern created by its mantra.

The most basic yantra form is a six pointed star, with the Shiva force as the upward pointing triangle and Shakti, the downward pointing one. These triangles are also forms of the linga and the yoni. The *Sri Yantra*, the most elaborate of the yantras, combines five downward facing triangles representing Shakti and four upward pointing triangles representing Shiva.

In a three dimensional form, the Sri Yantra is the cosmic mountain, *Mount Meru*, the central world mountain, and the mountain of the spine. In terms of light forms, Sri Yantra represents the Moon and the crown chakra, in which the higher union of Shiva and Shakti occurs, dispensing bliss to our entire being. It is this inner union of Shiva and Shakti that is the real goal of practice.

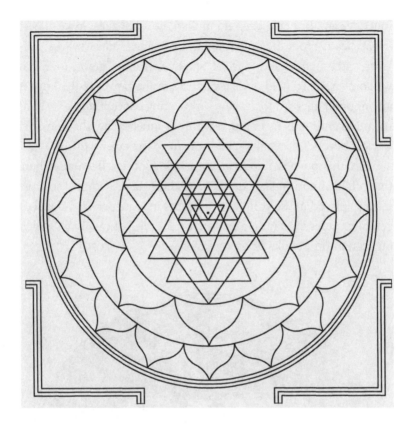

Yantras are present in the world of nature as the crystalline forms in minerals and in snowflakes. Fractile geometry reflects the vision of the yantra into mathematical terms extending through all that we see. The universe consists of a pulsating network of cosmic forces, of Shiva and Shakti energies, that create various geometrical patterns, through which all forms are structured. The universe is a great yantra of incredible power and intricate beauty that one can contemplate forever.

Meditative Experience of the Linga and the Yoni

The experience of the Shiva linga in yogic meditation is of a pillar of light, energy, peace and eternity, expanding the mind, opening the inner eye and bringing deep tranquility and unshakeable steadiness to the heart. From the crystal light of the linga radiate waves, currents, circles and whirlpools of Shakti spreading grace, love and wisdom to all. To hold one's awareness in the power of the linga is an important method to develop unwavering concentration. It calms the mind and putts us in touch with our inner Being, the immortal witness beyond the agitation and sorrow of the outer world.

For this purpose, you can find a Shiva linga from anywhere that offers Hindu puja or devotional items. Best is to get the linga form as placed in the yoni, which occurs in stone, crystal, metal or ceramic. At least pick up a picture or drawing of the linga, which one can find in books or on the internet.

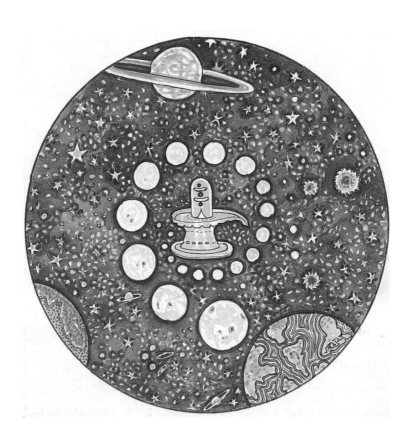

Visualize this Shiva linga with its circular yoni base in your heart and the conical linga extending up to your head, opening and steadying all the higher centers of consciousness within you. You can use the mantra **OM Namaḥ Śhivāya**, *to aid in this process, connecting to the Shiva energy behind all that is.*

Human sexuality is one of the many manifestations of the cosmic forces of duality, of a greater Divine sexuality as it were, which transcends all creaturely existence. We must learn to see the cosmic energy behind human sexuality rather than reduce spiritual symbolisms to our own physical and emotional inclinations. This is another aspect of Yoga in which we must look beyond our human psychology to the universal consciousness, if we want to transcend our creaturely limitations. Then we can see the dance of Shiva and Shakti as a Divine love of Spirit and nature through and beyond all dualities.

Unless one can meditate deeply upon the linga and the yoni as the dual Divine powers behind all existence, manifest and unmanifest, one has not yet developed a real understanding of Yoga. We must learn to discover the Divine union of the dual great cosmic powers in all that we can see or imagine.

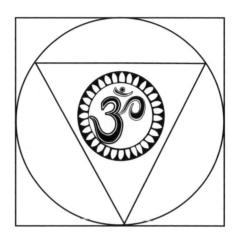

PART TWO

Working with the Universal Shakti

*Holding the entire universe through its pervasive nature that
has no form, the lightning of Shakti generates sound in the
Void, breathing its energy, and shines forth.
The Goddess is this lightning force by a subtle radiance. As the
Mother of all, she experiences all modes of being in the universe.*

GANAPATI MUNI, *PRACHANDA CHANDI TRISHATI* 235–236

This section of the book will examine Shakti as the cosmic power behind the forces of nature, the mind, emotions, and senses, and in the practice of Yoga. Various meditation techniques for working with Shakti will be explained, so that the reader can learn to work with Shakti in his or her own daily experience and moment by moment perception.

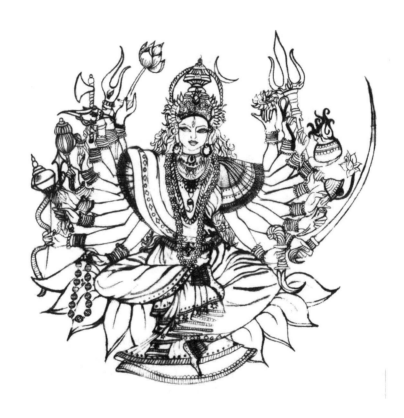

Mahadurga

The Primacy of Shakti

The ultimate goal of human life is liberation of the Spirit—called *Moksha* in Sanskrit—the realization of the Pure Self or Brahman beyond time, space and karma. In that Pure Self alone is complete and lasting freedom, peace and happiness. This highest truth is made clear in many great yogic teachings since the time of the most ancient *Vedas* to the great gurus of the modern era.

This supreme goal of pure unity is not hard to describe and the quest for it is something that we all know of in our deepest hearts, where we seek oneness with the entire universe. The important and difficult question that arises, however, is how can we get there? How can we reach the Supreme Self and Absolute Existence? That pure Self is so far removed from our ordinary experience that it requires a radical change of our entire way of life to even approach it.

The Absolute Brahman is devoid of qualities, beyond action and without any desire. It is extremely difficult to access even for those who genuinely have the sharpest minds and the purest life-styles. Brahman, moreover, is beyond all paths, unattainable by all efforts or by any striving. It is outside of time, space and causation and cannot be produced by any action. The very one who seeks it

53

must himself disappear before he can find it. Yet even having the thought of the ultimacy of Brahman does not take one there or even insure that one is going in the right direction!

Only if our minds can become fully concentrated within the heart can we know That Supreme Being. Those whose minds are clear and internally focused can certainly enter into the formless Brahman whenever they wish. But if there is any unfulfilled desire within us, we cannot reach it, or if we are able to touch it, we cannot abide in it. The problem is that we are full of desires, even if our minds are strong and subtle. Desire is the essence of all that we do and the very force behind our lives.

We do not live in Brahman, in the unmanifest beyond time and space, but in the manifest realm of life experience, filled with its energies, attractions, repulsions and attachments. In our ordinary minds and emotions, we are the products of time and space and cannot think outside of them. We are caught in place, person, form and karma as the very foundation of our personal and social reality.

We cannot go beyond this manifest realm unless we first recognize the power behind it. It is not within our personal capacity to go beyond the realm in which we exist, of which we are a creation. Only the power that has created this realm can take us beyond it. *So the real question is, what is the power behind the universe, behind our bodies and minds and how can we work with it to reach the Ultimate?*

The real power behind the manifest universe is Shakti, the energy of the Goddess, which is Brahman's force of expression, the Absolute overflowing itself into time and space. Shakti as the power of creation controls everything that occurs within her field. The formless Brahman beyond creation has no concern about this temporal realm or what we may do within it. From its point of view, there never has been any birth or death; there is no individual or cosmos, no bondage or liberation. Even our seeking to attain it has no meaning for it.

Our lives depend entirely upon Shakti, which grants us vitality, feeling and awareness, through which we set in motion both our outer actions and our inner spiritual practice. Shakti controls the entire manifestation, just as electricity allows all appliances to work. She rules over the processes of birth and death and the unfoldment of karma. She provides our souls with the bodies and minds and the worlds in which to experience life. All that we eat, breathe, perceive, feel or know consists of some portion of her energy, some aspect of her dynamic processes that surround us on every side. All that we seek to acquire for sustenance, happiness, knowledge or growth is part of her and derives from her.

Shakti also controls the way beyond manifestation, the return to Brahman. Even to seek Brahman, to look for what is beyond Shakti, we must work with Shakti. We must gain a special power and dispensation from her in order to do so. Shakti provides us the capacity for meditation and the discriminating insight through which we can transcend time and space.

The best means for both spiritual realization and for gaining all the goals of life is to worship Shakti, to work with and for the Goddess. There is no other way as effective, if there is any other way at all. *If Brahman is the goal, Shakti provides both the path and the power to traverse it.* We can awaken and follow her current to Brahman, or remain asleep under her outside streams that move in different directions.

Therefore, the issue is not Brahman, which is beyond everything, but Shakti that manifests everywhere. Shakti is all around us, flashing forth in all things, whether we recognize Her presence or not. The real issue is *how to gain the grace of Shakti*—How to ally ourselves with the right Shaktis in order to facilitate our development as an immortal soul.

We must recognize the primacy of Shakti or few if any of us can ever come to Brahman. Even great Yogis dedicated to the nondual Absolute worshipped Shakti as in the classical yogic text *Tripura Rahasya*. Or they had to recognize the importance of

Shakti, as in the case of Tota Puri, the guru of Ramakrishna, who even after his Self-realization came to worship the Mother.

Everything is controlled by Shakti. Shakti is closely connected to all that we depend on, all that attracts us and keeps life going and developing. Think about it carefully. Birth, reproduction and sexuality are all through Shakti, as the sexual power. Food and eating are another play of Shakti, as the power of nourishment. Breath, life (Prana), emotion and feeling are all owing to the Shaktis or vital energies which sustain them. The great elements of Earth, Water, Fire, Air and Ether are all forms of Shakti, which is their underlying energy. The prime gunas or qualities of Nature of Sattva, Rajas and Tamas are the root forces of Shakti. Our successes, gains, goals and achievements in any endeavor are only possible because of Shakti or the power of accomplishment.

Science and technology have developed many new methods of working with Shakti on an outer level, from electricity to nuclear power, that have transformed our external world order. The mass media is a play of Shakti in the field of communication, which has spread its network to every town and village on the planet. The Earth itself with its rich diversity of life forms is the biological field of Shakti, as the land with its energies, textures and ecosystems. The stars beyond are but the flashing forth of the cosmic Shakti through the unbounded expanse of space. Even subatomic particles are alive with powerful subtle forces of Shakti, which form the matrix out of which they dance.

All the things that we are attached to or involved with are forms of Shakti or are rooted in Shakti. Whatever we love, seek or desire is some aspect of Shakti that endows forms with color, beauty, charm and delight. It is not the object, person, place or experience itself that is the real source of our fascination but the energy, *rasa* or essence, which reflect the Shakti working through it. We are under the allure of Shakti in one way or another, whether we recognize it or not.

We cannot get beyond anything unless we first honor the Shakti behind it, which means to touch its core energy in consciousness. You cannot renounce anything that you are really attracted to, however hard you may try. But you can recognize the Shakti behind it and concentrating on it, move beyond the limitations of the form. This is like the bee that gathers the pollen and does not remember the form or shape of the flower from which it came. The Shakti within an individual object or an experience is ultimately the same Shakti throughout the entire universe.

We cannot get out of the realm of Shakti unless we recognize and honor the Shakti that is both in this realm and beyond—unless she decides. If she is not willing, our efforts will remain in vain. If she is willing, then we will be guided along the way and she herself will lead us forward. We can follow her flow and need no longer calculate or push our way onward, propelled instead by her grace. Yet for this to occur we must first learn to discover the movement of Shakti inside ourselves, which is the inner power of the soul to seek the truth.

Shakti is the way to the Godhead or Brahman. If you want to practice Yoga, you must awaken the Kundalini Shakti in order to take you forward. If you are devoted to God or the Goddess in any form, you must have that Shakti of devotion to lead you on. For any ritual, mantra or meditation to work, its Shakti must be first be invoked in order to give it power. Even Self-realization is only possible through the grace of Shakti and her *Buddhi Shakti*, or power of intelligence, through which spiritual discrimination works.

In that original Shakti there is no duality between the manifest universe and the unmanifest Absolute. It is the same Shakti in its active and inactive modalities. The Supreme Shakti holds the formless Brahman in the world of form, not by limiting it but as the overflow of her dance. Whether a devotee worships Shakti for home and happiness or for the highest liberation, it is the same Shakti on different levels that one is calling upon.

If you want to change the world through political action, you must first gain the Shakti or power to do so. Without that divine, integrative and transformative Shakti, whatever social reform or revolution is started will only end up in further conflict, violence and confusion.

If you want to be a great artist, you need the corresponding capacity or Shakti, the power and skill in that field of art. Everything has its characteristic Shakti, which contains not only the energy but the key to its manifestation like DNA, both the motivation and the energy necessary to bring it about.

So relative to whatever spiritual practices you may choose to do or whatever in life that you may seek; do not forget the primacy of the Shakti and you will never lose your way. The inner Shakti will gather all the outer Shaktis and take you to your true goal.

Shakti as the Cosmic Energy

The Goddess contains all the forces of both nature (Prakriti) and of the spirit (Brahman), of both the world of creation in time and space and the Absolute beyond all manifestation. All powers are rooted in *Parashakti*, the 'Supreme Shakti', the blissful energy of consciousness, *Chidananda*. It is through bliss that consciousness expresses itself and gives rise to all creation. This is not merely a philosophical statement but something we can experience inside ourselves. It is bliss or joy that motivates us at the deepest level of our being, without which we do not even want to stir!

Parashakti has many names and can be indicated by different Goddesses in their transcendent forms. She is worshipped as *Lalita* (she who plays), *Rajarajeshvari* (the queen of all the ruling powers), *Tripura Sundari* (the beauty of the three worlds), *Kamakshi* and *Kamakhya* (she who has lovely eyes), but also as Kali, Tara and Lakshmi. All the Goddesses are her manifestations.

The Supreme Shakti is *Chit-Shakti* or the power of consciousness which transcends and underlies both *Prakriti* (manifest nature and its processes) and *Maya* (the magical power of creation). Chit-Shakti, the power of consciousness, works through Maya as the power to envision, imagine and measure the world in the Cosmic

Mind. This Maya power unfolds itself into form through Prakriti, the process of nature and its inherent laws and rhythms through the gunas, elements and pranas, according to which both the worlds and living creatures are structured.[23]

Yet the power of consciousness itself also enters into the world as the hidden force behind the evolution of life and mind. Nature works according to a secret Shakti to develop matter into life, mind and intelligence, directing the soul by stages to its ultimate goal of Self-realization. In addition to this primary 'evolutionary Shakti', are specific 'developmental Shaktis', relative to the great forces of nature, from the many powers of the physical universe to those of the psyche. A living spiritual energy pervades and directs all things. If we open ourselves to its presence, we can discover beauty, wonder and delight everywhere!

The Goddess as Time, Space and Karma

Parashakti manifests through the three cosmic powers of time, space and action (kala, desha and karma). Most of us look at time, space and causation in an abstract manner as if these were mere concepts necessary to structure our experience. To look at them as forms of the Goddess may be difficult, but once we understand the universe as a manifestation of Pure Consciousness, we can easily do so. Time, space and action are the life, body and movement of the Supreme.

Kala Shakti means the 'power of time', which is personified as the Goddess Kali. The power of time has the capacity to create, sustain and destroy all things. It brings about birth, nourishment, growth, ripening, maturity, decline, decay and death. Its different facets manifest according to the ages, stages, phases and seasons of life. All life consists of an interweaving of the rhythms of time through creation and destruction, along with an inner growth and evolution of consciousness that continues through all outer changes of form in the spiral of Shakti.

The main way of reading the effects of Kala Shakti is through Vedic astrology, the science of time and light, particularly relative to mundane astrology (muhurta), which is the form of astrology used for judging the daily influences of the stars. Daily astrological influences or Muhurta, revealed through the Hindu calendar or *Panchanga*, indicate the forces of time operating at any given moment and how to best use their potentials. It is like an inner or cosmic weather report, one could say.

The best way to honor Kala Shakti among the Goddesses is to worship Kali, particularly in her form as the Eternal Mother. Time arises from the Prana or life-force of Shiva. The love aspect of Shiva's Prana creates Kali to guide us back to our source in the eternal. Kali's power works through time and its transformations, to take us beyond time to the timeless.

Desha Shakti is the power of direction or placement in space. Different locations in space provide not only a place of operation but constitute a particular realm of experience or *Loka*. The Earth itself is such a realm with its specific powers, qualities and influences relative to its mountains, valleys, plains and shores. The region on Earth in which we live is yet more specific with local variations of terrain and climate. More specific yet is the house we reside in, which has its own directional orientation and situation relative to the ground.

Vastu, the Vedic directional science, is the means of knowing the powers of location and adjusting our lives accordingly. Vastu shows us how to orient our houses, buildings and temples properly so that we bring in the best possible spatial influences and avoid those which can be harmful to our well-being.

Various Goddesses are related to space, most notably *Bhuvaneshvari*, the Goddess as the Queen of the worlds, the Goddess as the matrix of space which creates and rules over everything. Kali also represents the primordial space or womb of creation. Time creates space as its field of manifestation.

Karma Shakti is the power of causation through which events occur in the space-time continuum. Karma is inherent in both the movement of time and in the structure of space. Time is the movement of karma and space is the stage that karma creates on which to unfold its patterns. Time and karma are closely related, so the Goddess Kali has a rulership over both. She represents the desire from which our karma springs, which is ultimately the desire to realize the Absolute truth.

The Vedic birth chart (the 'Jataka' aspect of Vedic astrology), correctly read, shows how our karma is likely to manifest during the movement of our lives, from its primary potential at birth to its different expressions through various planetary periods or *dashas*. Vedic astrology also provides a means of altering karma, primarily through the worship of planetary deities, but also through the use of special planetary gemstones.

Ganesha is the deity who has the full knowledge of all karmas and also provides the tools to change them. Changing our karmas requires not only external factors like proper orientation in time and space, but our own actions of ritual, Yoga and meditation to bring us into harmony with the universal forces. In this regard, Ganesha is the main son of the Mother, the son of Shakti, who works to protect her forces and guide their manifestation. One should always remember Ganesha as the Lord of the universe and as the cosmic intelligence that projects the power of the Cosmic Mother. His elephant head carries all the wisdom and power of nature.

Shakti and Electrical Energies

As an energetic force, Shakti is referred to as *Vidyut-Shakti*, which literally means 'lightning', but indicates all the energizing electrical like powers of matter, life, mind and consciousness. Another Sanskrit term for lightning is *Tadit,* a common Tantric term for Shakti.

Light creates space as its field of activity and remains inherent in space as the potential of all other energies. The highest form of Vidyut is this universal energy hidden in space, only a small portion of which gets activated for the creation of the universe. It is from this original Vidyut Shakti of space that all other Shaktis arise. This transcendent lightning power sets in motion the Divine Word or **OM** vibration (Pranava) through which all processes in the universe are generated. It activates the life-force or Prana at a universal level. Its manifestation is the most beautiful and subtle display of scintillating flashes, weaving love and light into waves of ecstasy and grace.[24]

Lightning also manifests through clouds, not only rain clouds in the atmosphere but clouds of stars in space, the swirling of the nebulae. As electrical energy, lightning flows through water. As life-energy, bioelectricity, or Prana it flows through the water of the bodily fluids in creatures, the plasma and blood. Lightning is also hidden in the mountains or denser forms of matter, like the currents of force within the Earth and its magnetic field.

Many different forms of the Goddesses can be understood relative to the equation of Shakti and lightning. The Goddess is related to the cloud or mountain (with the cloud as the mountain of the sky), through which the lightning arises. As the 'daughter of the mountain', she is called *Parvati*.

Lightning is connected with the fall of rain and itself appears like a current or waterfall of light, bringing about a descent of grace from the higher planes. Water and river Goddesses, which are common in Hindu thought, reflect the lightning force in the waters. These include *Ma Ganga*, who symbolizes the lightning of the river of heaven, and *Sarasvati* who indicates the mountain lake of contemplation and the waters of the Moon.

We can identify the lightning aspect of Shakti with electromagnetism as a cosmic force and the root of all the powers of the universe. Parashakti is the supreme electro-magnetic force in operation in all things. Yet in doing so we are using the term in a broader and more symbolic sense than in modern physics. We are using it to refer to the attractive and propulsive forces behind all forces of body, life, mind and spirit.

Vidyut Shakti is the basic transformative and cataclysmic energy behind this magical universe. The entire universe is an artistry of the highest lightning in its multidimensional play and transformations. From the Big Bang that created the universe, to the formation of supernovas in the galaxy, to comets and meteors in the solar system, to hurricanes, tornados and volcanic eruptions on Earth, this lightning force is ever active, bringing about sudden changes that leave lasting marks upon the world.

This supreme energy of space is symbolized by the Goddess Kali, who governs over Shakti and relates to Vidyut or electrical energy. She is the lightning that arises from either the dark blue rain cloud or the dark blue expanse of infinite space. The electrical aspect of Shakti is activated at an inner level through her mantra **Krīm**, which has a stimulating and energizing effect on the mind and nervous system.

This prime electrical force is strong or even harsh in action, relentlessly keeping everything in the universe moving on track towards its goal. On an inner level, it creates awareness and perception, life and breath, though which a material body can become a conscious being.

Yet this original electrical energy also has an attractive aspect. The complementary magnetic aspect of Shakti is called *Akarshana–Shakti* or 'the power of attraction'. Besides magnetic forces, it is related to the power of gravity that holds the universe together, and to the power of love on a psychological level, which serves to unite all creatures.

The universal magnetic force is symbolized by the Goddess *Sundari*, the Goddess of beauty, love and delight—the bliss aspect of consciousness that draws everything back to itself. Her mantra,

Klīm, has an attracting and consolidating effect, magnetizing our nature to the higher truth and light. It is the balancing force in the universe that keeps the electrical energy from becoming too agitated or dispersing. It makes sure that the electrical currents of our lives gradually draw us back to our origin and goal in the Divine.

Akarshana Shakti holds objects in form as in the spherical shapes of the heavenly bodies and their ability to maintain their positions in space. It keeps us grounded in our bodies and minds and provides a continuity through the changes in our lives. It causes us to seek union with others and to integrate ourselves with our greater environment.

Yet these two forces or Shaktis (vidyut and akarshana) are one as electro-magnetism in the broader sense. Electricity creates magnetism through the polarity and duality by which it operates. We are naturally attracted to those people or events in which there is a greater energetic expression or movement. Conversely, magnetism creates an electrical force to draw things together. It is this action of unification, as in sexuality, that brings about the greatest electrical energy. The two forces are like attraction and repulsion, positive and negative charges, which depend upon one another and are ultimately one force in a dual manifestation.

The two mantras, **Krīm** for the cosmic electrical force, and **Klīm** for the cosmic attractive force, are also very close in form, differing only by a single letter. The letter-**Ka** indicates desire, action and prana. The vowel-**I** gives light, direction, motivation and energy. The difference between the two mantras lies in the semi-vowels. The semi-vowel **Ra** indicates the fire element and creates combustion, while **La** indicates the earth element and allows for cohesion.

Solar and Lunar Energies

Light is the dominant force in the universe and is related to electro-magnetism, which is the energy of light. From another perspective,

Shakti is twofold as the forces of the Sun and the Moon or solar and lunar energies, which indicate the broader powers of light as projection and reflection, not just the Sun and Moon as heavenly bodies.

Solar and lunar energies relate to the powers of the day and the night, which can stand for the light and dark phases of all time cycles. Daylight projects an activating and electrical force, propelling us to do things. Night creates a nurturing and attractive force, drawing us into a state of introversion and rest.

Solar energy reflects the electrical or active power of light and is warming, stimulating and motivating. Among the Goddesses, it is symbolized by *Bhuvaneshvari,* the Queen of the World, and her mantra **Hrīm**, which increases solar energy or the projective aspect of light.

Lunar energy reflects the magnetic or attractive power of light and is cooling, nourishing and calming. It is symbolized by the Goddess *Lakshmi* and her mantra **Śrīm**, which increases lunar energy or the reflective aspect of light.

Within the body, solar energy is the prana or the life-force that motivates and activates us. Lunar energy is the mind (manas) in the broader sense, our capacity for reflection, contemplation, feeling and attraction. Solar energy dominates the right side of the body and the flow of the breath through the right nostril, while lunar energy dominates the left side of the body and the flow of the breath through the left nostril.

Agni and Soma: Fiery and Watery Energies

Shakti is also twofold in manifestation as *Agni* and *Soma*, a concept that includes but goes beyond our ordinary ideas of fire and water, which these terms refer to outwardly. Agni and Soma indicate all prime dualities as sun and moon, electricity and magnetism, knowledge and devotion, and male and female. Generally speaking, fire is more electric and water is more magnetic, but the two also represent a greater densification of energy through the five elements.

On a higher level, Agni is the perceptive power of consciousness and Soma is its reflective power. Meditation consists of the dynamics between the two. Both Shiva and Shakti are *Agni-Somatmakam* or 'of the nature of both Agni and Soma' and have their fiery and water, harsh and soft or Agni and Soma forms. Agni and Soma are important as the root and crown chakras of yogic energy, holding all of higher awareness between them.

Soma like water is cooling, creative, nourishing, refreshing and revitalizing. Among the great Goddesses, it is symbolized by the Sundari, the Goddess of beauty and delight. Her mantra **Klīm**, which reflects the moistening power of water as well as the power of attraction, helps to develop the Soma within us. Another important mantra for Soma is Lakshmi's mantra **Śrīm**, which represents the light power of water, its ability to reflect, like the light of the Moon, which gives devotion and delight.

Agni as fire is heating, destructive, stimulating, activating and transformative. Among the great Goddesses, it is symbolized by Durga, the Goddess of protection and power, and her mantra **Dūm**, which functions like a forest fire to remove negativity. Perhaps the most fiery Goddess is *Bhairavi* and her mantra **Hsklrīm**, which represents a roaring fire or inferno in its movement from the depths to the heights. Agni can also be invoked by the Shiva mantra **Hūm**, which energizes the heat of Prana. This mantra also relates to various fiery Goddesses like Tara and Chinnamasta.

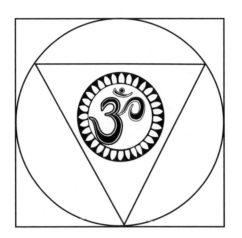

Meditation on the Shaktis of Nature

Nature fashions a complex web of marvelous processes in a vast array of activities on physical, biological and psychological levels. Whether it is the intricacy of the brain, the workings of subatomic particles, or the functioning of quasars, an infallible power and unbounded intelligence is present that is beyond our ability to calculate or even to conceive. Through the practice of the inner Yoga, we can learn how to work with this universal power 'from within' to transform the nature of our own consciousness from the mundane to the transcendent.

Yoga philosophy looks at the world of Nature according to the concept of *Prakriti*, which means the 'primal process, model or way of action', through which the cosmic order proceeds. Prakriti as the observable world order is contrasted to the *Purusha* or higher Self as the background observing consciousness. For this reason, there is a tendency to reduce Prakriti to something merely material, though it is much more subtle even than the mind which is its product.

Prakriti manifests through 'Cosmic Intelligence', called *Mahat Tattva* in Yoga philosophy, which is the first of her creations that unfolds the root energies, archetypes, qualities and elements according to which the worlds are structured. At a biological level, Prakriti evolves the bodies of living beings through the sense organs, motor organs and powers of the mind inherent in her energies. Prakriti has its own Shaktis or special powers on different levels, through which we can understand and master all of her processes.

The Shaktis of the Three Gunas

Prakriti consists of three *gunas* or 'prime qualities' of manifestation, which are the most fundamental energies that compose her. These are *Sattva*, meaning balance or light, *Rajas* indicating agitation or energy, and *Tamas* as inertia or matter. The universe consists of the interplay of these three gunas on various levels.

The gunas are not just abstract principles but contain the original powers of creation, preservation and destruction operative in the universe. The gunas are the most subtle and beautiful of all phenomena, the very essence of all energies, qualities, colors and principles. To touch them is to reach the very matrix of all creation and hold the potential to create all that was, is or ever could be—a profound mystical experience in itself.

The gunas are the most powerful forces at work both within and around us. Yoga requires that we recognize and honor them if we want to grow in consciousness. Each of the three gunas has its inherent power or Shakti (Guna-Shakti).

- *Sattva guna* as the quality of light has *Prakashana Shakti*, 'the power to illumine', which gives clarity and understanding to the mind, faith and devotion to the heart, balance and strength to the life-force, and purity and cleanliness to the body.
- *Rajo-guna* as the quality of energy has *Prerana Shakti*, 'the power to set in motion'. This power vitalizes the Prana, energizes the body, stimulates the mind and activates the

emotion, but in the process can cause disturbance, disequi-
librium and agitation.

- *Tamo-guna* as the power of form (or matter) has *Sthambhana
Shakti*, 'the power to resist or to stop'. This allows for the formation of the body, the holding the life-force and the mind in
the body, and the quieting of the emotions through sleep, but
can be a force of inertia, obstruction and resistance.

Through comprehending the Shaktis of the three gunas, we
can master all the forces in the universe. Developing Sattva as the
inner light of discrimination is the key to mastering Rajas and
Tamas. Yet we need the power of Rajas to break down the inertia
of Tamas, and the stability of Tamas to hold Rajas from becoming
overly agitated. Each guna has its place, though under the rule of
Sattva. Rajas is the creative force that sets things in motion. Sattva
is the balancing force that sustains things in action. Tamas is the
destructive force that brings things to an end.

The Goddess of wisdom, *Sarasvati*, represents the quality of
Rajas as the power of creation. *Lakshmi*, the Goddess of prosperity,
represents Sattva as the power of balance. *Kali*, the Goddess of
time, represents Tamas as the force that brings all things to an
end. Yet these are not the ordinary gunas that create bondage but
their higher forms (Para Sattva, Para Rajas, Para Tamas), which are
integrated into the working of Cosmic Intelligence as evolutionary
powers.

Meditate upon the Supreme Goddess according to these three
forms and functions. This is the best way to know and to use the
gunas.[25] Use the wisdom of Sarasvati to direct your energy of Rajas
according the dharmic principles of cosmic intelligence. For this
you can repeat her bija mantra **Aim**. Use the harmony of Lakshmi
to strengthen the quality of Sattva within you. For this you can repeat her bija mantra **Śrīm**. Use the power of Kali to remove the
darkness of tamas and its inertia. For this you can repeat her bija

mantra **Krīm**. Or you can chant all three mantras to the Goddess: **OM Aim Hrīm Krīm**, to transform the gunas within yourself.[26]

The Shaktis of the Five Elements

Yogic thought regards everything in the universe as a development of the five great elements of earth, water, fire, air and ether, which represent the different layers of manifestation from the subtlest spirit to the heaviest matter. The three gunas work through the five elements to form the outer world and to sustain the bodies of the individual souls that take birth within it.

Relative to Shakti, the elements indicate different degrees of densification of the underlying energy of consciousness. Each element consists of a particular vibratory state of energy which maintains a specific equilibrium of its own. The five elements have their inherent Shaktis and its various functions. These 'elemental Shaktis' (Bhuta Shaktis) are the source of the structure, complexity, texture and beauty of the objects that we perceive in the external world. They are the forces that uphold the forms and energies in the visible universe.

- Space has the powers to pervade, loosen, disintegrate and disperse. It holds the secret force of all the other elements. Space is the ocean of potential electrical energy, its inner lightning, of which everything in the universe is a reflection.
- Air has the powers to set in motion, to churn, agitate, stimulate, dry and desiccate. It represents the actualization of the electrical energy inherent in space, which manifests as various currents, clouds, nebulae, channels and wormholes.
- Fire has the powers to give warmth, cook, ripen and to impart color. It represents the electrical energy inherent in space, activated by air, becoming luminous and giving forth the powers of light.
- Water has the powers to cool, moisten, nourish and to adhere. It represents entropy of fire as heat is lost and turns

cold. It has its own currents, denser than air, which can hold fire, air, electrical force and ultimately life-energy itself.

- Earth has the powers to support, to carry, resist and to sustain. It holds the other elements hidden with itself as its special spaces (caves), water, fire (at the core of the Earth), and air (gases within the Earth).

The Shaktis of the five elements can be worshipped as forms of the Goddess as the Earth Goddess, Water Goddess, Fire Goddess, Air Goddess and the Goddess of Space. When we recognize the Shakti of each element, we move beyond its outer form to its inner power. When we recognize the Goddess ruling each element, she will unfold its secrets for us.

All the Goddesses have connections with the five elements as one aspect of their manifestation. They can represent one element or principles that work with more than one element. Most commonly, the Goddesses relate to the feminine elements of space, water and earth, which serve to hold and contain. But the Goddesses have their fiery and airy forms as well.

Meditation on the Shaktis of the Elements

Meditate upon the Shakti of the elements and forget their outer forms. Look to the energies of the element rather than to the objects composed of them. Following this procedure, let your awareness move beyond the outer world of objectivity and enter into the inner universe of Shakti where all appearances dissolve into currents of consciousness.

Meditation on the Shaktis of the Earth Element

Look upon all objects made of Earth as manifestations of the creative capacity of the Earth element. Forget about the differences between these objects made of Earth and concentrate on the creative power of the Earth element as their essence.

Learn to recognize the underlying power behind the different objects made of Earth in terms of shape, form, density, weight, permeability, color, size, resistance, and support.

Hold the essential energy of the Earth element within you, particularly at the Earth or root chakra, using the bija mantra for the Earth element **Lam**. Be one with all transformative Earth energies in the universe. Feel the teeming forces of the Earth within you from the powers that build up the mountains, to those that make the oceans, to those that sustain life in the soil.

Mediation on the Shaktis of the Water Element

Look upon all phenomenon made of water as manifestations of the creative power of the Water element. Forget about the differences between the forms of water as rivers, ocean, rain, ground water, ice, waves or currents and concentrate on the creative power of water as their essence.

Learn to recognize the underlying power behind the different properties of water as coolness, dampness, cohesiveness, nurturance, and oiliness.

Hold the essential energy of the Water element within you, particularly at the Water or sex chakra, using the bija mantra of the water element **Vam**. Be one with all transformative water energies in the universe. Feel the teeming forces of Water within you from the waves of the ocean, to the currents of the rivers, to the falling of the rain.

Meditation on the Shaktis of the Fire Element

Look upon all phenomenon made of fire or light as manifestations of the creative power of the Fire element. Forget about the differences between the aspects of fire as heat, light and color or its forms as fire, sun, moon or lightning, and concentrate on the creative power of Fire as their essence.

Learn to recognize the underlying power behind the different properties of Fire as heat, dryness, the power to ripen, digestion and transform.

Hold the essential energy of the Fire element within you, particularly at the navel or Fire chakra, using the bija mantra of the fire element **Ram**. Be one with all transformative fire energies in the universe. Feel the teeming forces of fire within you from the fires on Earth, to the lightning in the atmosphere to the Sun and stars in the sky.

Meditation on the Shaktis of the Air Element

Look upon all phenomenon of air as manifestations of the creative power of the Air element. Forget about the differences between the forms of air as wind, clouds and currents, or it's various movements as expanding and contracting, ascending and descending. Concentrate on the creative power of Air as their essence.

Learn to recognize the underlying power behind the different properties of Air as lightness, dryness, coldness, movement, and stimulation.

Hold that essential energy of the Air element within you, particularly at the Air or heart chakra, using the bija mantra of the air element **Yam**. Be one with all transformative air energies in the universe. Feel the teeming forces of air within you, from the currents of the wind in the atmosphere, to the solar wind, to the forces that propel the galaxies.

Meditation on the Shaktis of Space

Look upon all objects that exist in space as manifestations of the creative power of space. See form and structure as but a force field existing within space and pervaded by space. Look at all objects in space as united by space.

Another method is to concentrate on the space between objects and forget about the objects. Try to hold your power of seeing in the power of the presence of space. Look at space as the reality and the objects in space as just temporary formations or crystallizations of the energy of space.

Hold the essential energy of the Space element within you, particularly at the throat or space chakra, using the bija mantra of the element of ether **Ham**. Be one with all transformative energies of space in the universe. Feel the teeming forces of space within you, from the caverns in the earth, to the expanse of the atmosphere, to endless potentials of the space within and beyond the stars.

Mediation on the Mind Space as the Sixth Element

Space is not simply external but also exists internally. As a practical means of experiencing this, first go to a spacious external place, like a broad open field, where you can look out on the distant horizon. Then internalize that expanse of the horizon as the space within your own mind. Close your eyes and imagine that same expanse existing within you.

Hold the essential energy of the mind space within you, particularly at the third eye, using the bija mantra of the mind space **Kṣam**. Be one with all transformative energies of the mind, pervading the universe in the space of the mind. Feel the teeming forces of mind within your inner space, from your own thoughts, to those of all living beings, to those of the Cosmic Mind.

Meditation on the Space of Consciousness as the Seventh Element

Consciousness has its own space. Yet while the space of the mind is a space of thought and sensory perception, consciousness has an objectless and thought-transcending space.

Expand your inner consciousness into the infinite void that is prior to and beyond the appearance of any objects, conditions or experiences. Let all thoughts dissolve and fade away into it.

Hold the essential energy of the space of consciousness within you, particularly at the crown chakra, using **OM**, the mantra of the supreme space. Let your mind open up beyond the boundaries of your head into the infinite space beyond. Be one with all transformative energies of consciousness, sustaining the universe as the supreme space. Feel the teeming forces of consciousness within your inner space, above and beyond all manifestation, holding the seed potential of all that could ever exist.

The Shaktis of the Five Subtle Elements Or Sensory Qualities (Tanmatras)

Besides the gross elements are corresponding subtle elements, the five sensory qualities of sound, touch, sight, taste and smell. Sound is the subtle element or sensory component through which we can know the element of space. Touch is the subtle element or sensory component through which we can know the element of air. Sight is the subtle element or sensory component through which we can know the element of fire. Taste is the subtle element or sensory component through which we can know the element of water. Smell is the subtle element or sensory component through which we can know the element of earth.

Called *Tanmatras* in Sanskrit, the subtle elements are the root energies behind our sensory impressions that give vitality and meaning to them. They are the essences (rasas) derived from our sensory experiences, which reflect the pleasure or pain, beauty or disgust, happiness or sorrow, spiritual elevation or depression that we gain from them.

The Tanmatras, like the Gunas, are not just abstract concepts but powerful forces, which artists and yogis understand at a deep level of inner vision. Each has its own Shakti or characteristic power. The subtle elements build up our subtle, astral or energy body, which consists of the residues of our physical experiences. It is this body that we continue with after death and which becomes the vehicle for deeper yogic practices.

The Subtle Element of Sound

The power of words, sounds and music to stimulate, heal or bring peace is well known to all of us. We spend most of our time speaking, listening to others speak or listening to other forms of sound and music. The sound tanmatra creates the environment and an atmosphere for our thoughts and our moods, forming the background and support for all that we do.

Through working with the Shakti of sound, we can raise our awareness and level of energy. Learn to focus on the 'sound behind the sound', as it were, striving to hear not just particular sounds but to hear sound itself in all of its possibilities. Look for the essence of music, rhythm and tonality in all that you hear. Try to hear the energy behind the sound, the silent point within from which the sound arises, and not just the sound itself. One way to do this is to go out in nature and try to connect the sounds that arise with the expanse of the sky as their origin and goal.

The Subtle Element of Touch

The power of touch based impressions to transmit life, love, warmth and affection is the basis of personal intimacy. It is an important factor in healing through therapeutic touch and massage. Touch can give life energy, as when we embrace another, or can harm life, as when we strike another. The touch tanmatra is the strongest and most intimate of the sensory potentials in its affects, coloring our feelings and desires. It transmits the Shakti or energy of the person directly, for good or ill.

Through working with the Shakti of touch, we can raise our awareness and level of energy. Learn to focus on the 'touch behind the touch', as it were, striving to feel not just particular touch sensations but the underlying ability to touch in all of its possibilities. Look for the essence of feeling in all things that you touch. Try to touch the energy of pure feeling behind different touch sensations, from which the sensation of touch arises, and not just the sensation of touch itself. Another way to do this is to remember your breath or prana as you touch things.

The Subtle Element of Sight

The power of sight based impressions, particularly color, is well known for healing, spiritualizing and energizing effects. The colors around us stimulate our mind and prana and affect our moods and thoughts. The sight tanmatra brings light into the Prana and mind, connecting us to all forms of vitality. It is the most powerful Shakti of the senses for awakening the mind.

Through working with the Shakti of sight based impressions, we can raise our awareness and level of energy. Learn to focus on the 'scene behind the scene', as it were, striving to perceive not just particular visual sensations but the background screen of light on which they are all projected. Look for the essence of light in all that you see. Try to see the energy of light rather than the objects that appear in it. Be one with the light of seeing as the basis of all that you perceive.

The Subtle Element of Taste

Taste based impressions have a power to stimulate the appetite, move our prana and link us together at an emotional level. This is another matter of common experience, as various family dinners, restaurant gatherings and communal feasts indicate. The taste tanmantra has the power to awaken our taste either for the higher or the lower things of life, and to condition our feelings in one direction or the other. Life is about the cultivation of taste. This depends upon what we desire in our hearts.

Through working with the Shakti of taste, we can raise our awareness and level of energy. Learn to focus on the 'taste behind the taste', as it were, striving to not just perceive particular tastes, but to grasp the taste of bliss behind all the flavors of life. This is to look for the essence of taste in all that we experience as pure delight. It is to become aware of the taste of life, nature and the universe itself.

The Subtle Element of Aroma

The power of aromas to calm the mind, as in the use of incense and aromatic oils, or to beautify us with different perfumes, is another important enhancement in our lives. The smell tanmatra awakens the mind and senses and nourishes the heart. It creates our subtle environment or the subtle Earth around us.

Through working with the Shakti of fragrances, we can raise our awareness and level of energy. Learn to focus on the 'aroma behind the aroma', as it were, striving not just to sense particular aromas but to grasp the aroma of life itself, which is the incense of the soul. This is to look for the essence of aroma in all that we smell. Learn to contact the fragrance behind all that you contact in life, the subtle residue that it leaves on the soul.

The Cosmic Form of the Goddess

The Goddess holds the universal subtle body made up of the cosmic tanmatras or subtle elements that are the essence of all experience. The Goddess is the essence of all sound, touch, sight, taste and smell sensations possible in their Divine energy, origin and majesty. She is the ultimate power of beauty and delight behind all the impressions that our senses are able to bring in. Her form is the most amazing display of music, color, fragrance, flavor and touch, not as mere bodily sensations, but as currents or waves of beauty and ecstasy pervading the entire universe. To touch the body of the Goddess, which is beyond all physical and mental forms, is to experience the entire world as Brahman, the Absolute.

Meditate upon the essence of all beauty in the universe, whether of earth, water, fire, air or ether, whether of smell, taste, sight, touch or sound, whether of name, form or action, animate or inanimate as flashes of the dance of lightning of the Supreme Goddess. Be one with that endless and eternal play of lightning that is ever weaving a dance of bliss through the space of consciousness.

Meditation on the Shaktis of Body and Mind

One of the most important and transformative methods of meditation is to meditate on Shakti as the prime force behind all dualities. In this practice, one focuses on Shakti as the power linking both subject and object. Concentrating on that power as the true reality, one gives up both subject and object, and merges into the Shakti beyond all duality.

Whether it is the power of thinking, seeing, feeling or just being aware, the underlying power is one and derives from the Supreme Shakti. That power is formless, of the nature of energy only, and is not limited by the subject or objects that it serves to connect. That power, moreover, is not inanimate but the very force of consciousness that is the presence of the Goddess. Tracing back all energies to the Supreme Shakti at their origin, anything we do can become a means of liberation of the Spirit.

In this 'meditation on Shakti', we merge into the flow of Shakti which pervades all things and provides them the energy with which to function. Shakti is both the executive (decision-making) and instrumental (administrative) power in the universe. From this supreme power, all dualities arise as different polarities, as its positive and negative charges. We can follow these connections into a greater network of unity beyond the boundaries of objects, sense organs or individuals.

Meditation on Shakti is one of the main yogic methods taught by Ganapati Muni, the chief disciple of Ramana Maharshi.[27] It combines the observational approach of the Yoga of knowledge with the recognition of Shakti as the supreme principle. *Meditation on Shakti is the pursuit of Shakti from the standpoint of the Yoga of Knowledge (Jnana Yoga).* In this regard, we can start with the Shaktis or powers through which the mind operates.

1. The Shaktis of the Mind

The mind is an incredible energy field, with a rapid movement of impulses and connections, creating an elaborate information network and synthesis of ideas. Even the most elaborate computers yet developed today cannot approach this. The mind has a tremendous though subtle power that can hold innumerable details, memories, names, calculations and opinions. *The mind, we could say, is Shakti's greatest creation in the manifest world.* Through it we can interact with the universe around us as part of the fabric of our own being that has no limitations.

In these meditation practices, one concentrates on the Shaktis or powers behind the different functions of the mind as thinking, feeling, memory and self-sense. These correspond generally to the yogic classification of the mind as *buddhi* (intelligence), *manas* (emotional and sensory mind), *chitta* (memory) and *ahamkara* (self-sense or ego).

Meditation on the Shakti of Thinking (Vichara Shakti)

Thought is the basis of our entire mental activity, whether of an intellectual, emotional, sensate or instinctual content. The mind itself is nothing but a bundle of thoughts, strung together by the power of memory.

Real thinking or deep deliberation, however, is a higher level of conscious thought that relates to our 'inner intelligence' or *buddhi* in yogic practice. This higher intelligence comes into play when we seriously ask fundamental questions in life and search out, through deep examination and observation, the inner truth of things, a process that is called *Vichara* or 'inquiry' in Sanskrit.

To practice this meditation on the Shakti of thinking, focus on the power behind the thinking process and forget about either yourself as the thinker or the ideas that you can think about. Look on both the thinker and the thought as manifestations of the greater power of thinking which is universal in nature.

Inquire, "What is the power through which I can think and where does it come from?" Trace the power of thought back to its origin in the deeper awareness in your heart. Recognize that your power of thinking is a manifestation of a universal force like electricity and not something that belongs to you personally.

If everything can be thought about, then everything is intelligible and everything ultimately is thought. What is the mental power that creates and sustains the entire universe in all of its intricacy? Try to link your self to the power through which everything is thought, but which itself cannot be limited to any particular thought.

Meditation on the Shakti of Feeling (Chetana Shakti)
Feeling is the underlying mood, tone or color of the mind in which thought occurs. Feeling is more enduring than thought, which changes every instant. Feeling is more subjective than thinking and usually more engaging. It occurs when we bring ourselves into our perception and experience. Feeling involves pleasure or pain, joy or sorrow, peace or agitation. It is never neutral like thinking. Its highest expression is bliss or *Ananda*.

In this meditation on the feeling aspect of the mind, focus on the power of feeling and forget about the one who has feelings or the objects that one has feelings about. Look upon both the one who feels and the objects felt as manifestations of the deeper power of feeling which is universal in nature.

Inquire, "Where does the power of feeling arise from and what is its nature?" Recognize that your power of feeling is a manifestation of a universal force like electricity and not something that belongs to you personally. Try to merge into that primal power of feeling which is life, love and delight at its core.

Another method is to try to understand the power of feeling that underlies all our emotions, whether desire, fear, anger, love or hate. It is the intensity of feeling that makes an emotion important and allows it to make a mark upon our minds. Try to live in that intensity of feeling or passion and give up the external objects and events that may trigger it, or the particular emotions that hold it. In the pure intensity of feeling we can let go of all particular emotions and understand the basic energy of feeling that is the grace of the Goddess.

Meditation on the Shakti of Memory (Smarana Shakti)
Memory is the ultimate result of our mental activity. The power of our memory reflects the strength of our awareness and attention. Through the power of memory we can understand the complete movement of time and karma within our minds. Cultivation of inner memory or Self-remembrance is the essence of meditation.

In this meditation, focus on the power and presence of memory and forget about you as the person who remembers things or the particular events you might remember. Look upon both the one who remembers and the events remembered as manifestations of the underlying power of memory, which is the power of awareness to endure and support all things.

Meditate upon where memory comes from inside you, where it resides and what is the power that sustains it. What is the power within us that can link the past, present and future events? How can that which has no form hold such innumerable forms through the process of time?

Cultivate your power of memory with sustained concentration. One of the best ways to do this is to practice Self-remembrance, to strive to remember the inner Self or Divine presence in all that you do. Another way is to remember a certain mantra like **OM** or **Hrīm**. Hold to it in the background of your mind as the root of your memory and concentration.

One can also strive to daily remember a great truth principle or great spiritual teacher. Another way is to continually hold in mind the Devata, the God or Goddess that one worships. In all that we do we are cultivating one form of memory or another. Let us make sure that the memories that we cultivate are like flowers that render a sweet fragrance for all time.

Meditation on the Shakti of the Sense of Self (Ahamkara Shakti)
Our sense of self or I-thought is the primary thought behind all the activities of the mind on all levels and of prana itself. From its energy arises the motivation for all that we attempt to do in life. The ego has a tremendous power invested into it, both in terms of memory and life-force. If we learn to hold to that power, we can let go of the ego, and redeem its energies as well.

In this meditation, focus on the power of self-being and forget about either the self or the other. Look upon both the self and the other as manifestations of a greater power of self-being. Learn to contact the self-sense or sense of self-being that underlies the activities of all the five senses and of the mind itself.

For this, first remember that it is only because oneself exists that one can pursue other subjective or objective activities. Inquire into the ground of your own being, the power that sustains you and links together your ordinary activities. Follow out the great inquiry, "Who am I?" which is the most important of all the pursuits of human knowledge. Cultivate the power of self-awareness and self-being within you. Let your 'I' expand to embrace all that exists.

2. The Shaktis of the Senses

Each of the five senses has its inherent Shakti through which it functions. These color our minds and emotions and influence all that we do. How we use our senses determines whether our actions are karmically harmonious or disharmonious, whether they bring us peace and joy or agitation and suffering.

In Vedic thought, the senses are the Gods (Devas) that rule over us and can elevate our consciousness if we approach them in a sacred manner. We must learn to use the senses well, with respect for their particular Shaktis that are part of the Divine Shakti.[28]

Each sense has its unique capacity and power. The ears have the power to grasp sounds, the skin to feel touch, the eyes to see light, the tongue to taste and the nose to smell. The senses allow us to recognize the gross and subtle elements (sense potentials) which relate to them: the ears with sound and space, the skin with air and touch, the eyes with sight and fire, the tongue with taste and water, and the nose with smell and earth.

The sense organs develop and evolve out of the seed Shakti of feeling. They are our mind's instruments to know the external world and to imagine the internal world as well. Besides the gross sense organs in the physical body are subtle sense organs in the mind, which have no outer form. These subtle senses allow for higher perceptions and even what is called 'extrasensory perception', like seeing or hearing at a distance.

The senses are sophisticated transmitters of powerful energies from the external world, affecting us at intimate levels at every moment. They are the main source of the external influences that dominate most of what we do. To master the senses is to master the entire world. The key to mastering the senses is to gain control of the power that moves them, the Shakti within then.

Most of us today, live in urban environments with little contact with nature and engage our senses with media based impressions that are one-dimensional and artificial in nature. It is important that we take the time to liberate our senses in the world of nature, where we can experience real depth perception, variety of colors, subtle sounds, an array of fragrances, and all the other dimensions of experience which requires that we contact the greater universe around us. This natural yogic liberation of the senses is necessary for the liberation of the deeper mind and heart. By meditating upon the Shakti of the sense organs, particularly in the world of nature, we can develop acuity of the senses and extend the range of the senses into the subtle and supernormal ranges.

In this practice, one meditates upon the Shaktis or powers behind our sensory functions while letting go of the likes and dislikes that arise through sensory contacts. The senses, after all, are only instruments. What is the power that allows them to function, just as the electrical source that allows various machines and appliances to run? That power is much more important and determinative than the instrument itself.

In the process one of focusing on the Shaktis of the senses, one turns the senses within. Their outgoing activity is replaced with an ingoing energy or Yoga Shakti. This internalization of the senses increases sensory acuity as well, allowing them to reflect the light of consciousness within and reveal to us the Divine nature of all that we perceive.

Meditation on the Shakti of Seeing (Drishti Shakti)
The sense of sight is the most important of our senses. It is an essential tool for all higher Yoga practices. The sense of sight relates not only to the physical sense but to deeper perceptive powers of the mind and heart. We can follow the same method with both the inner and outer powers of seeing.

In this meditation, focus on the power of seeing and forget about either the seer or the seen. Look at both the seer and the seen as manifestations of the underlying power of seeing. It is the state of seeing itself that subjectively becomes the seer and objectively becomes the forms that are seen.

Another method is to practice *Shambhavi mudra*, which consists of directing one's attention within while looking at objects externally. Hold your gaze within while the eyes remain open. An aid in this process is to visualize a flame in the center of the spiritual heart, and remain connected to it in whatever else you are sensing or doing externally.

Yet another way is to focus on the space between objects and not look directly at the forms of the objects themselves. Regard all objects as creations of space, which outlines them. And look at the power of space as the power of perception. A good way to begin this meditation is to look at a tree but focus on the space between the leaves and branches, rather than the leaves and branches themselves.

One can focus on light itself as the power behind both the seer (light as an instrument of perception) and the seen (light as an object of perception). Hold to the power of light and let go of the objects seen. Be one with the light of seeing.

Meditation on the Shakti of Hearing (Shruti Shakti)
The sense of hearing relates not only to the physical body, but to deeper powers of the mind and heart to be receptive and to comprehend higher truths. Through it we can open our consciousness to direct knowledge and communication. We can follow the same method with both the inner and outer powers of hearing as with the sense of sight.

In this meditation, focus on the power of hearing and forget about either the hearer or the sounds heard. Look at both the hearer and the heard as manifestations of the power of hearing. It is the state of hearing that subjectively becomes the hearer and objectively becomes the heard.

Another way to do this is to listen for the silence between each sound. This will lead you into hearing yet more subtle sounds.

You can extend the practice further into searching for the silence between each thought. Look at the waves of sound as a manifestation of the ocean of silence, which holds the highest power of hearing and listening.

Yet another way is to focus on hearing the natural sound of the breath as **So-ham**, with 'so' as the sound of inhalation and 'ham' as the sound of exhalation. It is the power of the sound of the breath that allows all sounds and words to manifest. Try to remember the sound of the breath as you speak through the outgoing breath.

A final method is to place your mind in the space of hearing and let its sphere expand with all the sounds that you hear. Follow the sound current into the Infinite.

Meditation on the Shakti of Touching (Sparsha Shakti)

The sense of touch, is not just an external potential, but relates to the ability to be touched generally, including at an emotional level. Touch has perhaps the strongest Shakti of the sense organs, as it affects us most intimately and personally. It works mainly through the skin that serves to define the boundaries of our physical body.

In this meditation, focus on the power of touch and forget about either the hand that touches things or the objects that are touched. Look at both the skin and the objects and energies felt as manifestations of the power of touch, which brings energy and vitality to the entire body.

There is an electrical current through which the sensation of touch is transmitted. We feel this current more acutely with stronger sensations of pleasure and pain or of heat and cold. Try to follow the energy of touch that is behind pleasure and pain and let go of the pleasurable or painful objects in the mind. Trace the energy of touch to the energy of life and feeling in the universe. Learn to use your inner hand to touch all that is.

Meditation on the Shakti of Tasting (Rasana Shakti)

The sense of taste has its subtle counterpart as our ability to develop taste in what we do or imbibe. Taste connects us to the *rasa* or the essence of things. It relates to speech, which also occurs through the tongue, as the expression of taste.

In this meditation, focus on the power of taste and forget about either the tongue that tastes things or the food items that are tasted. Look upon both the tongue and the items tasted as manifestations of the underlying power of taste.

A good way to do this is to try to taste the Prana or life-force in food or beverages, their underlying vital energy. Hold to the 'taste of Prana' and let go of the food items which carry it. See how the Prana derived from the sense of taste energizes our vocal organs, stimulates our appetite, and awakens our vitality overall.

At a deeper level, strive to develop the power of taste in all that you do, looking to the deeper qualities in things, as opposed to their mere sensate value. Try not merely to develop taste in an aesthetic or artistic sense but in a Yogic sense, learning to imbibe the 'flavor of Ananda' or bliss behind all our sensory impressions.

Meditation on the Shakti of the Sense of Smell

The sense of smell, like that of touch, is intimate and personal. It is connected through the nostrils with the breath and is the power of the breath to feel things at an instinctual level.

In this meditation, focus on the power of the sense of smell and forget about either the nose that smells things or the objects that are smelled. Look upon both the nose and the objects its smells as manifestations of the power of the mind to grasp aromas. Become one with the aroma and forget about yourself or the objects from which various fragrances arise.

A simple way to do this is to use incense during meditation. Sandalwood is traditionally considered the best in yogic thought owing to its calming purposes, but many others are also good.

Merge the mind in the aroma of the incense and behind that in the power of the sense of smell which is able to recognize the aroma.

Or take a fragrant flower and meditate on where the fragrance comes from. It arises quickly like an electrical impulse. What generates it within you? What is the root of all fragrances in the mind? Let your life be like the fragrance of the flower. Let there be a Divine fragrance that emanates from your entire being.

3. The Shaktis of the Motor Organs

The motor organs, like the voice, hands and feet, are powerful forces that drive us, expressing strong instinctual, emotional and sensory impulses. As powers of action, they rest upon our desire and will power.

In these meditation practices, one applies the same methods as with the sense organs. One looks to the power that allows the organs to function and ceases to be concerned about their particular activities. Yet while the sense organs are knowledge-based, the motor organs are action-based, so their energy is easier to work with.

Meditation on the Shakti of Speaking

Speech is the most important of the motor organs and the driving force behind all our expressions. To control speech is to control both the mind and the prana. To accomplish this, we should focus on the power behind speech, which ultimately links us up to mantra and to the Divine Word.

In this meditation, focus on the power of speech and forget about either the one who speaks or the details of what is said. Look upon both the speaker and what is spoken as manifestations of the greater power of speech. It is the power of speech that subjectively becomes the speaker and externally becomes the words that are articulated.

A good way to do this is to focus on the current of sound out of which speech arises. Try to follow the sound current within you back to its source in the inner heart. Note that the power of speech manifests out of the power of the breath, when the breath is linked to the power of the mind. For speech to occur, the mind must work with the breath through the process of exhalation, projecting the outgoing air through the vocal organs.

Another method is to hold to a bija mantra like **OM** and merge all other words, sounds and meaning into it. **Aim** is probably the best mantra in this regard because it is the power of Divine speech. Become one with the power of the mantra and forget both yourself and the world.

Meditation on the Shakti of Strength in the Hands
The hands represent the universal function to grasp, to hold and to make. It is this cosmic power of grasping that one should try to understand, whether in your own hands, those of another; the hands of other creatures or their different types of organs of grasping and holding.

In this meditation, focus on the power that allows your hands to function and forget about functions and movements of the hands. Look upon both your hands and what they grasp as manifestations of the cosmic power of grasping.

Try to feel the strength that you have in your hands by tightening them in the form of a fist. See how the muscular power of the hands connects to the greater strength of the body and further to the will power of the mind. Try to link your personal strength with the well springs of cosmic energy in your awareness. Become one with the 'hand of light' which fashions all the worlds.

Meditation on the Shakti of Movement in the Feet
The feet manifest the universal power of movement, which occurs through different organs and powers of movement. Everything in the universe is in motion in one way or another.

In this meditation, focus on the power that allows you to move your legs and forget about either the legs or where you are going with them. Look upon both the feet and the places you may move to as manifestations of the power of movement, which pervades all space.

Recognize the power of movement that you have physically in your legs and see how it reflects your greater vitality. See how it connects to the greater powers of movement in the universe, starting with the vehicles that you use to travel, and culminating with the motion that pervades the universe through the stars.

Let your bodily movements enter into the universal movement and with the great Shakti that allows the universe to unfold its endless dance. Let every step you take be an arrival into the Infinite.

Meditation on the Shaktis behind the Reproductive, Urinary and Excretory Organs

Our urinary and excretory organs are lower aspects of broader cosmic functions to work with the water and earth elements. Reproduction is the creative aspect of this function, while elimination is the purificatory side of it.

In this meditation, focus on the power that allows you to remove water through the body by the process of urination. Do the same with the power of excretion. What is the source of the impulse from which urination and other vital urges arise? It is a pranic urge, much like an electrical impulse. From what point does that impulse enter into the conscious mind? Where does that energy remain in potential when these vital urges are not active? Learn to contact that pranic force.

Going further, inquire what is the power that sustains our internal organs, like the stomach, intestines and liver, which have no outer actions? Try to connect to the universal power of Shakti that operates the organic processes of the body and keeps them so marvelously regulated.

Relative to the power of reproduction, recognize the energy of creation in all the procreation that occurs in the universe. Learn to hold to that creative energy and let go of the forms that it creates. Let that creative energy renew both your body and your mind.

4. The Shakti of Prana

Shakti has rhythms of ascending and descending motion, expansion and contraction, inner and outer impulses. These constitute the 'breath of Shakti' which is the life of the universe. Once the Shakti awakens within us, her breath and currents of vital energy will unfold these movements and make the body move according to their impulses as part of the cosmic dance.

The main form of Shakti or functional energy that we have within us is that of Prana or the vital force. *Prana is the guiding Shakti of both body and mind.* It is not only the root power but reflects a secret intelligence found that works behind both instinct and superconsciousness. Prana is most active in the motor organs but also allows the senses to work and, at a deeper level, provides the impetus for thought and emotion. All the Shaktis of body and mind are 'Shaktis of Prana'.

Prana is the Goddess within us. Our life-energy and its impulses come from the universal Shakti and are a portion of her manifestation. *Worshipping Prana as Shakti is perhaps the highest form of worship* in which life becomes a sacred ritual and thought itself becomes prayer and mantra. Our life belongs to the Goddess. Our blood belongs to Kali, as it were. This recognition of the Goddess energy awakens the Kundalini Shakti within us and enables our entire life to become a Yoga practice and a spiritual adventure.

Meditation on Prana Shakti

In this practice, we emphasize the Prana or vital energy behind the various aspects of our nature. We hold to that primary power and let go of what the mind and the senses may perceive or do, as but an expression of it.

- First, relative to mental processes: hold to the energy behind the mind, the power from which thoughts arise, that is connected to the energy of the breath. Learn to 'breathe with your thoughts' and let your thoughts rise and fall like clouds moving quickly across the sky.
- Second, relative to the sense organs: hold to the energy behind the senses, the power through which the senses function, that is connected to the energy of the breath. Learn to 'breathe through your senses' and let your sensory impressions rise and fall like clouds moving quickly across the sky.
- Third, relative to the motor organs: hold to the energy behind the motor organs, the power through which you are able to use them, that is connected to the energy of the breath. Learn to move your body along with the breath. Note that most exertion occurs through the outgoing breath. The energy belongs to the breath, not simply to the motor organs which are but instruments.

We can also work Prana directly through the breath, through the practice of pranayama or yogic breathing. *The practice of pranayama is perhaps the best way to work with the power or Shakti of both body and mind.* All pranayama practices have their relevance here. We will just mention a few of the most important.

First is a meditative form of pranayama. For this, focus on the power of the breath and forget about either inhalation or exhalation. Look upon both inhalation and exhalation as complementary aspects of the power of the breath. Try to merge your awareness into the power of the breath and where it arises from, like the ocean from which the waves come.

Another method is to simply observe the breath, holding to the power behind the breath, letting inhalation and exhalation move naturally without interference. One can use the mantra 'So-ham' along with the processes of inhalation (**so**) and exhalation (**ham**).

Another method is to follow the current of inhalation as a cooling force up the spine to nourish the mind and senses, and to follow the current of exhalation as a warming force down the spine as a means of energizing the power of speech and the motor organs. Try to become aware of the pranic currents within you. Recognize all the pranic forces that move within you as manifestations of the Supreme Shakti.

An advanced method is to meditate upon the Shaktis of the five forms of Prana: *Prana* as the inward moving propulsive energy centered mainly in the head, *Apana* is the downward moving energy of elimination centered mainly in the lower abdomen, *Samana* as the equalizing force dwelling mainly in the navel, *Vyana* as the expanding energy working mainly in the heart and chest, and *Udana* as the upward moving energy working mainly in the throat. One should learn to be able to direct the prana in all these five ways.[29]

Shaktis of the Practice of Yoga

Classical Yoga is a development of the internal energy of consciousness, not simply a learning of outer forms of exercise. It draws us to the Inner Yoga of mantra and meditation as the primary practices. It does not stop short with the outer Yoga of asana and Yoga postures, though these are very helpful, if not indispensable, in preparing us for meditation.

Yoga is classically defined in the *Yoga Sutras* of Patanjali, the main traditional compilation of yogic principles, as the neutralization of the *vrittis* or 'fluctuations' of the deeper mind and heart, called *chitta* in Sanskrit.[30] Yoga can also be defined in a positive manner as the 'development of the Shakti, the spiritual power of awareness', through which the mind or chitta is naturally brought to a state of rest. In this regard, the *Yoga Sutras* also speaks of liberation in its last Sutra as "the power of consciousness (Chiti-Shakti) resting in its own nature."[31]

Yoga aims at reducing the disturbed and fragmented energy of the mind, while increasing the calm, concentrated or unified power or Shakti of pure consciousness. Yoga rests upon the *Yoga Shakti* or 'power of Yoga,' which is the energy, grace and action of the Goddess within. This in turn reflects the 'consciousness of Yoga' or the Shiva power of awareness, observation and detachment.

97

Shaktis of the Eight Limbs of Yoga

Each of the eight aspects or limbs of classical Yoga has its own Shakti on which it depends for its proper development. Each aspect is a stage in the deepening of the Shakti or power of consciousness. To really practice Yoga is not merely to outwardly conform to some outer practice, but to awaken the internal energy that naturally makes our entire life into Yoga. Entering into the flow of Shakti helps unfold Yoga from within, according to the needs and capacities of our particular nature and temperament.

1. Yama Shakti

Yama Shakti is the power or capacity to practice the five yamas or yogic observances of non-violence, truthfulness, control of sexual energy, non-stealing and non-possessiveness (ahimsa, satya, brahmacharya, asteya and aparigraha). These constitute the basic life-style principles and values behind all true Yoga practices or 'the universal ethics of Yoga'. Yama Shakti provides the power of self-control on which Yoga rests, which is the capacity to direct our will inwardly through closing the outgoing movements of prana, mind and senses.

To possess Yama Shakti within us means to be able to master our vital impulses and turn them into drives for spiritual perfection. All true power begins with the conservation of energy, through which energy can grow to a higher threshold of transformation. This is the role of the Yamas in Yoga. Yama Shakti is the power of yogic values.

2. Niyama Shakti

Niyama Shakti is the power or capacity to practice the five niyamas of self-discipline, self-study, surrender to the Divine, purity and contentment (tapas, svadhayaya, Ishvara pranidhana, saucha and santosha). Niyama Shakti is the steadying power of a disciplined life-style through which we can sustain our efforts along the yogic path for as long as we live.

To have Niyama Shakti is to maintain a yogic life-style that sustains an inner flow of energy and awareness behind all that we do. The self-discipline developed under the yamas leads to a change of behavior under the niyamas, in which our daily actions are imbued with consciousness. The niyamas constitute the real yogic life-style and Niyama Shakti is our ability to lead this, not merely through our own efforts but by contacting the cosmic powers within.

3. Asana Shakti

Asana Shakti is the power through which we can hold the body in various asanas or yoga postures without physical or mental strain. Asana Shakti is the power to rest comfortably in a single posture without internal friction. It turns all asanas into a natural seat for meditation, in which we easily forget body consciousness and naturally move within.

To possess Asana Shakti is to be able connect to the energy behind the form of the asana, in which the mind and prana naturally become calm. It does not mean achieving the perfect outer form of the asana, but using the asana as a conduit to allow the Shakti flow within us. Each asana has its own particular Shakti, through which its energy is released. These are reflected in the heating and cooling, expanding and contracting energies according to which the asanas are performed.[32]

Merge into the Shakti of your favorite asana and forget about yourself as the performer of the asana or your body as the form of the asana. Let that Shakti lead you on to further asanas or to just resting in stillness. Be one with the inner flow.

4. Prana Shakti

Prana Shakti is the power developed through the practice of yogic breathing or pranayama. It is a higher or deeper Prana that can be internalized to energize or to heal the body or mind.

To have Prana Shakti means to be able to calm the breath naturally, not through the effort of the mind or ego, but through linking our individual Prana with the cosmic Prana. It is learning to breathe with the entire universe as part of the breath of God. Each type of pranayama has its own Shakti or energetics through which it affects the Prana within us in different ways way.[33]

Hold to the Prana Shakti within you and let your effort to control Prana relax. Follow the flow of Prana Shakti and through it learn to breathe with and through all existence.

5. Pratyahara Shakti

Pratyahara Shakti is the power to internalize the energies of the sense organs, motor organs, prana and mind. This 'Shakti of internalization' provides the foundation for inward concentration and meditation, as the primary practices of the Inner Yoga.

To have Pratyahara Shakti means to be able to direct our energy inward at will. Through it we can turn around the movement of the prana and senses from the outer to the inner. Without this decisive inward turning of energy, our Yoga remains external and cannot bring about deeper realization. To develop this Shakti, learn to turn your senses off at will by developing a deeper aspiration within yourself. Learn the power of non-action and abide in non-doing as the source of all energy.

6. Dharana Shakti

Dharana Shakti is the power to sustain the focus of the mind in a consistent manner. It is most easily defined as 'the power of attention'. Whatever we give our attention to becomes energized and gains importance for us. Lack of attention, on the other hand, keeps us weak, dependent and confused in life.

Dharana Shakti consists of generating a steady stream of attention like the flow of a powerful river that carries away everything in its course. To have Dharana Shakti is to be able to concentrate the mind at will, just like the pointing of a light, and hold it comfortably on the object of concentration for as long as necessary.

We can best develop it through learning to fix and hold our gaze, as the eye is the power behind the mind. Dharana Shakti is the 'seeing power' of the deeper mind.

7. Dhyana Shakti
Dhyana Shakti is the power to hold the mind in a state of deep meditation. It is a natural force of peace and calm in the mental field, which opens and relaxes the mind at a deep level. Dhyana Shakti consists of holding the mind quietly in a receptive and reflective state, like a calm mountain lake.

To have Dhyana Shakti is to be able to meditate naturally and at will, whatever the circumstances around us or whatever we may be examining with the mind. Yet different methods of meditation will produce their particular types of energies and have their own characteristic Shaktis. Inquiry-based meditation approaches (called *vicharas* in Sanskrit), have the greatest power to awaken our higher consciousness and have the strongest Shakti of all meditation methods.

To develop Dhyana Shakti, cultivate the power of the mind to abide in stillness and space. Let the mind rest in its own formless nature, which is one with the Shakti of awareness.

8. Samadhi Shakti
Samadhi Shakti is the power of unitary consciousness to neutralize all negative karmic tendencies and put an end to all emotional suffering. It is the ability to merge the mind into the object of perception, so that the mind's movement no longer interferes with our process of seeing.

To have Samadhi Shakti is to be able to find the Divine bliss, beauty and delight in all that we experience. It is the highest power of Yoga, through which we gain the fruit of Yoga as oneness with all that we perceive. In samadhi, we merge into the ocean of Shakti. We let all energies merge back into the supreme Bliss of Being. To develop Samadhi Shakti, learn to merge your awareness into the deepest aspirations of your heart and be one with all.

Prana as Yoga Shakti

Overall, the power Prana is the main Shakti or power of Yoga. The Prana Shakti of Yoga allows us to have interest, enthusiasm, devotion and energy in our Yoga practices, whatever they may be.

The Yogic practices of right attitude and right action (yama and niyama) allow us to gather a spiritual prana in life. Asana is meant to remove negative tension and turn the body into a fit receptacle to carry the higher prana. Pranayama serves to develop the higher prana, while pratyahara functions to internalize it so that we can use it as a spiritual force. Dharana enables us to concentrate this higher Prana in the mind. In dhyana, the mind reflects the higher Prana beyond itself. In samadhi, the mind merges into the higher Prana in its cosmic source of pure awareness.

To develop your Prana as a Yoga Shakti, bring the awareness of Yoga into all your daily activities. This means to act according to the unitary rhythms of life and Being. Let your life be Yoga in communion with the universal Life.

Shaktis of the Different Branches of Yoga

Yoga is not one thing. It is an 'integral approach' to life and awareness. Therefore, Yoga has many definitions depending upon its level and manner of application.

Yoga can also be defined relative to different types or the main classical approaches to Yoga. These can be simplified into four major groups, which reflect the four main aspects of our nature, each with its own Shakti or inner power. To follow these paths of Yoga requires awakening the Shakti that can unfold it for us from within.

- The Yoga of Knowledge or Jnana Yoga: *Buddhi Shakti*, the power of inner intelligence, insight, discrimination and detachment.
- The Yoga of Devotion or Bhakti Yoga: *Prema Shakti*, the power of Divine love, devotion, beauty and surrender.
- The Yoga of Service or Karma Yoga: *Samkalpa Shakti*, will power, the power to work, and to accomplish one's deeper motivations.
- The Yoga of Energetic Practices or Kriya Yoga: *Prana Shakti*, the power of Prana and Kundalini.

True Jnana or spiritual knowledge rests upon Buddhi Shakti, the power of the higher mind to discern the true from the false, the eternal from the transient, the real from the unreal, or light from darkness. Buddhi Shakti is best developed through the process of meditative inquiry called *Vichara*, particularly in the form of Self-inquiry, pursuing the great inner quest "Who am I?". Other practices like study of spiritual texts, repetition of mantras and concentration exercises help in the process. One can also meditate upon the Goddess *Sundari* as the beauty of spiritual knowledge and seek her grace along this yogic path.

True devotion rests upon the awakening of the Prema Shakti or power of Divine love within us. Real devotion is not an egoistic emotion. It does not serve to promote one guru, sect or religion versus another as the only truth. It arouses the innate power of Divine love inherent within our souls. The best way to do this is through chanting the names and mantras of our Ishta Devata or the form of the Divine most dear to our hearts with deep devotion. One can also meditate upon the Goddess *Lakshmi*, particularly in her form as *Radha*, as the personification of Divine devotion.

True service is not simply doing what others tell us to do. It rests upon the strength of our will power, our ability to take a task upon ourselves and complete it, to not quit or waver until the goal is reached. The best way to develop this is to do our work with the fullest concentration but surrendering to the Divine. One can also meditate upon the Goddess *Durga* as the personification of the Divine will to protect, save and transform the world.

Truly energetic Yoga practices require an awakened Prana within us, which is a life energy attuned to the cosmic life and the universal breath. The best way to do this is through the practice of pranayama or yogic deep breathing, aligning our individual Prana with the cosmic Prana and the inner deity. One can also meditate upon the Goddess *Kali* as the personification of the cosmic Prana beyond birth and death.

The Shaktis of the Five Koshas and Seven Lokas

Yoga recognizes the existence of five *koshas*, sheaths or encasements of the embodied soul (Jivatman). Each has its own Shakti or functional power. The soul is the central presence (linga in Sanskrit), around which these Shaktis operate.

Each kosha corresponds to a certain *loka*, a world, level or plane of experience. Beyond these five are the two principles and realms of *Sat* and *Chit* as Being and Consciousness, which constitute the nature of the Self.

1. *Annamaya Kosha* or 'food sheath'—*Anna Shakti*, the power of food and nutrition and the power of the physical body to digest food through the digestive fire. It relates to physical matter, the physical world and the deity of Agni or Fire.

2. *Pranamaya Kosha* or 'breath sheath'—*Prana Shakti*, the power of breath and vital energy, the capacity for exercise, skill and strength of the motor organs and good instincts. It relates to the subtle energy field between the physical and the astral and the deity of Vayu or Wind.

3. *Manomaya Kosha* or 'sheath of the outer mind'—*Samkalpa Shakti*, will power and the power of determination, as also acuity of the senses, power of imagination, and good mental expression. It relates to the subtle or astral world and the deity of Soma or the Moon.

4. *Vijnanamaya Kosha* or 'sheath of the inner intelligence'—*Buddhi Shakti*, the power of intelligent cognition, the ability to reason, discern, discriminate and ascertain what is eternal, real, authentic and true (Satya Buddhi). It relates to the formless realms of higher meditation and the deity of Surya or the Sun.

5. *Anandamaya Kosha*, 'bliss sheath' or sheath of the inner heart—*Ananda Shakti*, power of love and bliss, the ability to imbibe the essence of beauty and delight from the diverse experiences of life. It relates to the higher realms of cosmic creation, the causal realm and the deity of Akasha or space.

6. Chit—the realm of Pure Consciousness—*Chit Shakti*, the power of consciousness and awareness. It relates to the plane of pure consciousness, to the Self or Atman as the deity.

7. Sat—the realm of Pure Being—*Sat Shakti*, the power of Being. It relates to the plane of pure being, to the Absolute or Brahman as the deity.

Ascending through these cosmic Shaktis, we move into deeper levels of the universe, manifest and unmanifest. Our current society has learned the power of energy and information, but remains ignorant of the higher powers of intelligence, bliss, consciousness and being, that are much greater and more profound. Learn to contact and set in motion all these Shaktis within you.

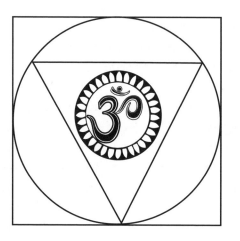

The Shakti of Relationship

Shakti is the power to link things together, the essence of which is relationship. Energy flows between things when they are magnetically aligned. The universe consists of a network of incredible, many leveled, multidimensional and interpenetrating energy fields in rapid motion, oscillation and transformation. This living fabric of relationship constitutes the cosmic organism.

The energy grid of our body links us to the energy field of our greater natural environment, the earth and air, through our biological processes of eating and breathing, as well as through our bodily movement in space. The energy grid of our mind links us to the greater field of the collective mind, through both external forms of the media and information and internal forms of feeling and thought. Through intuition and deeper perception, our mental pattern links us with the cosmic mind and the forces of intelligence that pervade all space. The universe of Shakti is a single unified yet infinitely variegated field of energy, where the One is in All and All is in the One, as a vortex of forces ever spiraling into itself.

Wherever there is Shakti, it serves to link us with something beyond our ordinary state and extends our boundaries. Through harnessing a few physical Shaktis, modern technology has allowed us to travel farther and faster on land and in space, to gain more information, and to reach a much greater range of sensory experiences. Yogic technology—through harnessing the deepest Shaktis of the psyche, of the mind, heart and prana—can allow us to travel beyond time and space, to know the truth directly beyond all information, and to experience reality more vividly than all that the senses can ever know.

The Power of Relationship

Perhaps the strongest Shakti in the human world is the Shakti of relationship and the power of association. Relationship creates the strongest bonds in life at physical, emotion, mental or spiritual levels. Relationship defines who we are through our self-image, personal expression and the social role that we play.

People have more energy, more Shakti in relationship, when their forces are linked together. By themselves, in isolation, their energy tends to become low or even depressed. In relationship, one's prana has a counterpart or partner who can reinforce and magnify it. Even along the spiritual path we benefit from the association of teachers and fellow disciples to increase our aspiration and dedication.

Relationship is the strongest force of bonding for human beings. It is much like the bond that exists between electrons and protons in the atom. Starting out with relationships between individuals, this force extends to the family, community, country, human beings in general, all life on Earth, all life in the universe and ultimately to the Supreme Self beyond all time, space and manifestation. To follow the universal network of relationship back to the Self of All is an important practice of Yoga and Tantra. Tantra itself literally means a thread, a fabric or a web, referring to the web or Shakti that forms the inner lines of force which sustain all things in the universe.

This means that we should be very careful about the type of Shakti we are creating in our relationships, starting at the level of personal intimacy where this energy is most poignant. Is the energy of our relationships a spiritualizing force, promoting the inner growth of awareness, or a materializing force, promoting desire and attachment? Is it a creative and nurturing force or a destructive and debilitating energy? Does it make us more kind, intelligent, aware and independent or more bitter, fearful, clinging and dependent?

We are creating energy patterns in our relationships that have important karmic implications for our soul. The emotions generated create deep-seated samskaras or karmic tendencies within us. Unless we understand and heal our associations, we will carry their negative patterns for the future and repeat them again and again.

It is an interesting fact that people have different chemistries in relationship, often above and beyond their individual potentials for good or ill. Some combinations of otherwise good people can be harmful and destructive. They simply don't mix. The reasons may be astrological, karmic or accidental. Other people can harmonize together even when there are significant differences in their physical, emotional, mental or spiritual affinities or makeup.

Sometimes we have what could be called 'fatal attractions'. We are attracted to and may bond with those who are not good for us at an inner level. There is in all of us a certain seeking of drama or rajo-guna in relationship that can get us addicted to the wrong people, just as it can get us addicted to drugs.

At the same time, there are divine connections in relationship. We have karmic affinities with certain individuals, connecting and communicating with them easily at a deeper level, almost as if preordained. The patterns of relationship are complex and mysterious. We must yield where the inner attraction exists but must break with outer attractions that take us downward.

Bhakti Yoga, the Yoga of Relationship with the Divine

Bhakti Yoga is the Yoga of relationship with the Divine, with the Devata within. It is probably the most important aspect of Deity

Yoga. Bhakti Yoga requires that we make our primary relationship not with others outwardly but with the Divine internally. It generally follows an 'emotional attitude' or *Bhava* to the Divine as father, mother, love, friend or master, using a particular form.

Deity Yoga is a 'Yoga of inner relationship', with the Deity becoming the prime focus of one's emotional attention. One learns to relate to the Deity as if to another person. One strives to relate to the Deity through all of life, seeing the face of the Deity in the sky, their form in the mountains, and their energy in the movement of wind or water. Through the power of devotion one can commune with the consciousness of all beings and all existence as one's own.

Yet this Yoga of relationship can be brought into our human relationships as well. It is the basis of the old Vedic dictum to treat one's father, mother, guru and guests as God. It is not a denial of human relationship but provides the basis for its spiritualization.

The Power of Association

The 'power of association' is well known to all of us for good or ill. What we do in company has more vitality to it and is easily magnified. This power is called *Sanga-Shakti* in Sanskrit, which extends to the power of the community and the power of society. The proper unfoldment of the individual depends upon a supportive social field or community. Meanwhile, the enlightened individual strives to create a sanga or society of awakened individuals to carry on their yogic work in the world.

Many special communities have arisen out of the power of association, whether it is a business community, a community of artists or a spiritual community. We naturally form groups, tribes, families, and societies based upon the structuring power of relationship.

The yogic deity governing this power of association and community is *Ganesha*, the 'lord or leader of the *ganas*', meaning groups or community. Every community has its leader, guide, prime mover and protector, its Ganesha. This Ganesha may be the guru, president, or CEO. Such an empowered leader should act according to dharma in order to selflessly provide for the welfare of everyone.

There is also the related tradition of *Sat-sanga* or 'association with the wise', as the association with spiritual teachers and gurus, which can be done formally or informally. When people come together around a teacher their inclinations and capacities to learn and grow spiritually are greatly increased. This reflects a deeper level of association that one could call 'the Satsanga of the heart'. It consists of emulating spiritual beings, powers and principles at the level of the spiritual heart. It is an important way to connect to the Guru, who may not always be physically accessible or even physically alive.

Such an 'inner attitude of communion' is an important way to connect to the Devata, particularly the Ishta Devata, the special form of the Divine one has chosen for worship. It is a key method for developing Shakti, particularly the 'magnetic force of Shakti', the *Akarshana Shakti* that draws Divine grace into us and allows us to bring it into others as well. When our life force and attention is magnetized inwardly by the power of Divine association, then the currents of Shakti are released within us and our awareness can spread its wings in all directions.

We must learn to use the power of relationship to develop a higher Yoga Shakti. If our relationships are superficial, they will create a lower Shakti that draws us into further desire and sorrow. For such higher relationships to occur, our inner heart must align itself with the highest Shakti that we can project.

The best way to do this is to emulate the relationship of Shiva and Shakti in our associations. We must center ourselves in the power of Shiva, or inner awareness, as the focus of relationship, and allow the full freedom of Shakti as creative intelligence to express itself. Relationship should be based upon a spiritual purpose (Shiva) but with an inner freedom, grace and delight (Shakti).

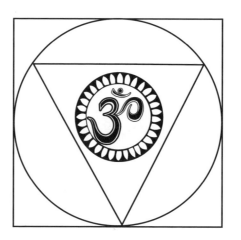

The Shaktis of Emotion

Emotions are the most powerful forces in our ordinary lives. They are the main form of Shakti that we must learn to harmonize in order to find any last peace or real happiness. Emotions are the keys to our inner and outer well-being.

Negative emotions can cause outbursts like lightning, waves or thunder that can catch us unaware, shocking and overwhelming us. They can throw us into disturbed moods that may last for days or years, upsetting our inner equilibrium in a fundamental way. They can affect our deeper thought patterns and our outer biological urges, triggering physical and psychological disease and making it harder for us to relate to our environment.

Positive emotions, on the other hand, are the strongest healing forces for body and mind. Kind words from another, expressions of affection and friendship or shared experiences of joy bring positive vitality and a better mood into our minds and hearts, uplifting us in a quick and lasting manner. Positive emotions can remove fatigue and toxins from the body, eliminate blockages and traumas from the mind, and elevate our overall functioning in life, making us more creative and spiritual. Love itself is the strongest of all transformative forces, not only for healing but for elevating our being to its heights in the inner Yoga.

The Tantric approach is to focus on the power behind a phenomenon, rather than its outer form as its true reality. Tantra looks at the energy behind the emotion as the most important factor, not the outer events or circumstances that might trigger it. As manifestations of cosmic energy, all things that exist are sacred and eternal. Energy can move in various ways; it can be changed, but it can never be destroyed. In this regard, each emotion possesses its own energy or Shakti, which is a manifestation of vital energy or Prana. This means that we cannot destroy a negative emotion but we can change a negative emotion into a positive emotion, and ultimately merge all emotions into peace, contentment and bliss (Ananda).

We can learn to work with our emotional energies just as we have learned to handle outer energies like electricity, fire or wind. Different emotions provide different challenges, but all emotions can prove difficult because emotions are invested with energies that are more primal than thought—a kind of instinctual power that can hold a strong ego focus as well. The intellectual mind cannot master emotion for this reason; a deeper feeling and awareness, moment by moment, is required for this to happen.

The Shakti of Anger

The Shakti of anger is particularly difficult to deal with because anger easily externalizes itself as an attack on someone or something. Anger arises as a defense mechanism deep inside us, so that we cannot easily question its validity.

Anger is a development of the self-protective instinct; its ego content is strong and automatic. Anger, one could say, is the self defending itself. Because of its instinctual power, our anger drives us to aggressive action, leading us to personal conflict and even causing wars at a collective level.

Recognizing the danger of anger, which is like a raging fire if we let it develop, helps us maintain detachment from it when its power arises. Honoring the fire of anger as a Divine force enables us to remove our personal identification with it. This requires that we have an inner fire of discrimination that does not blame others but takes responsibility for our own karma and motivates us to our spiritual quest as our main goal in life.

The following meditation on the Shakti of anger can also help us to deal with it: "There is no one who is angry and no person or event that one is angry about. There is only the force of anger as a cosmic power. Honor the power of anger as a universal energy of life and withdraw your personal involvement with it, and it will subside into pure vitality."

The Shakti of Desire

The Shakti of desire is also very hard to deal with because it is deep-seated. Desire is the basis of our embodied existence, the very root of the mind. We are largely a bundle of desires, shifting and changing at every moment, never at rest or content. We can be easily manipulated by an appeal to our desires or by the creation of artificial wants, which is what the commercial world is so adept at doing.

Desire is originally a force of imagination. To control desire we must first be in control of our power of imagination. Yogic methods of mantra, visualization and concentration are helpful for this purpose, which use the power imagination as a force for spiritual development. Visualizing the form of your Ishta Devata or chosen deity is a good way to do this.

Practicing deep introspection to discover what we really want in life is another method. What we all most deeply desire is inner peace, Divine love, and unity with all. This 'recognition of the true wishes of the soul' that are eternal can free us from the grip of the transient desires of the ego.

The following meditation on the Shakti of desire can also help us to deal with it: "There is no one who desires and nothing desirable in itself. There is only the force of desire as a cosmic power that stimulates all creatures into action. Honor the power of desire as a spiritual force and desire the highest for yourself and for everyone, letting go of all lesser wants."

The Shakti of Fear

The Shakti of fear is one of contraction, hiding and self-defense. This also makes it very difficult to approach, much less to change. Fear arises when we feel attacked or threatened, particularly when pain is created or our life is in danger.

All fears are based upon the fear of death. To really deal with fear is to face the fear of death. The world we live in is always uncertain, with death as a constant companion. Honoring death as the inner teacher is an important way to do this. Meditation on death is another method. Worshipping the Goddess Kali, who represents the eternal life beyond death, can help us in this regard. It is from the idea of a second entity, someone apart from or opposed to ourselves, that fear arises.[34] When we recognize that the entire universe is one with our deepest Self, the very ground for fear disappears.

The following meditation on the Shakti of fear can also help us to deal with it: "There is nothing other than my true Self in the entire universe. There is no one who is afraid and nothing to fear. There is only the force of fear as a cosmic power. Honor the power of fear as a universal energy of life and withdraw your personal involvement with it, and it will subside into pure vitality."

Emotions as Cosmic Powers

One of the best ways to work with emotions in Yoga is to honor all emotions as Devatas, forms of the Gods and Goddesses. For example, if we are angry, we can consign our anger to *Rudra*, the wrathful form of Shiva, to transform. In this regard, it is important that we do not project any thought of harm upon the person we may be angry with. We must surrender to anger as a Divine force and let our personal anger go.

If we are caught up in desire, we can look to beautiful forms of the deity, like the Goddess *Sundari*, and offer our personal desire to her. If we are afraid, we can call upon *Durga*, the protective form of the Mother Goddess to help us, who keeps her children safe from all difficulties and dangers, including death itself. Or we can call upon *Rama*, who is the form of Vishnu that protects all living beings from fear and distress.

Another way is to look at emotions as merely roles or attitudes of the mind, much like an actor does, and learn to play with them. In the traditional dramas of India, actors and actresses cultivate the emotions, *bhavas* or *rasas*, like fear, desire, anger, disgust and joy, learning to wear them like masks that our Prana wears in its dance of life.

One must be able to understand all the colors of emotion without being dominated by them. To do this one must first recognize and face emotion, not as a mere personal force but as a cosmic power. If we surrender to the Divine Shakti behind emotion then all emotions can be transmuted into light and energy healing to the heart.

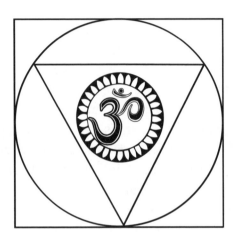

Healing Shaktis

Shakti is the great power of spiritual, psychological and physical well-being. Connecting to it, we can work wonders in healing ourselves and healing others, even from severe diseases and imbalances. By going directly to the source of the universal healing Shakti, we can move beyond the limitations of all outer therapies and drink inwardly at a fountain of boundless vitality and energy.

Each thing in the universe possesses its own special healing power or Shakti. Ayurvedic medicine teaches us how to recognize and work with these different healing Shaktis in its various therapies. Yoga must also consider their roles for any Yoga therapy to be really effective. In this chapter, these healing Shaktis are outlined, which could be an entire study in its own right.

The Atmosphere or Sphere of Shakti

The atmosphere is the dominant sphere of Prana, the realm of the global vital force through which the planetary organism functions. The term 'atmos' in atmosphere derives from the Greek term for breath that relates to the Sanskrit term Atman, which is not only breath but the Spirit as well.

The forces of the atmosphere—what is called the sphere of the wind or *Vayu Mandala* in Vedic thought—are responsible for the weather and seasonal changes that drive the movement of life on the planet. The atmosphere is the very breath of the planet, which grants life to all creatures!

Atmospheric forces and their weather patterns are the primary factors in the outer world for health and well-being. Our ability to adjust to their daily and seasonal changes determines whether we resist or succumb to infectious diseases starting with the common cold and extending to plagues and epidemics. Atmospheric forces convey the powers of heat and cold, dampness and dryness, wind and sunlight that make their mark upon our body and its energies. They create the outer environment, to which our inner environment or bodily state must harmonize itself in order to maintain balance.

Each one of us can be said to be a manifestation of the atmosphere, incarnate as an individual being, which exists as the breath within us. Living creatures are atmospheric forms that move along the planet's surface like the winds. In addition, we have our own 'inner atmosphere', our emotional and energy sphere. How we adjust to it through our moods, is essential to our psychological well-being.

The lightning in the atmosphere reflects the vibrant Shakti or life-force of the Earth, holding the solar energy in the clouds, which bring the rain that nourishes all living creatures. *The atmosphere is the great sphere of Shakti on Earth* with its dramatic storms and shifting clouds that move quickly on a daily or even hourly basis. Without the dynamic flow of air through the atmosphere, life would not be possible even for a minute.

Today, as we pollute the atmosphere, we are disturbing the flow of Shakti on the planet, which is like playing with lightning. This must have eventual destructive consequences as it upsets the bioelectrical currents of nature. The recent global increase in hurricanes, droughts and floods indicates the possible calamities that such an interference with the root of nature's power can bring about. If we severely disrupt the Shaktis of nature, we can set in motion forces that are beyond our control and may eventually threaten the very existence of civilization as we know it.

We must learn to work with the Shaktis of nature rather than against them. For this to be really possible, we must first recognize and honor these forces of nature as the Shaktis or Goddesses that they really are. A good way to do this is to perform rituals, mantras and prayers for the Earth Goddess, *Bhumi Devi*, in our Yoga and healing practices. We should also honor the great Goddess *Durga,* who represents the protective and saving form of the Mother working through all of nature.

The Healing Shaktis of Plants

The healing powers of the atmosphere enter into plants primarily through the rain. Plants, both as foods and herbs, are our natural healing substances, carrying the fluid of life and light.

Foods have their special healing and nutritive potentials and powers or Shaktis. These are reflected not just in the bulk constitution of specific food items in terms of sugars, fats and proteins, but also in their subtle nutrients of vitamins, minerals and enzymes. At a deeper level, it includes the prana that they carry and the love with which they are prepared.

Though their nutritive power is less, herbs have stronger healing Shaktis than foods. This is reflected in their therapeutic powers to promote sweating or urination, to remove cold or fever, to stop bleeding, to promote the healing of wounds or to facilitate rejuvenation, to just list but a few of their many capacities.

The Shaktis of foods and herbs rests mainly on their energetics as defined in Ayurvedic medicine as taste, heating or cooling affect and long term effect upon the digestive system, as well as other special properties.[35] A good Ayurvedic doctor knows the healing powers and properties of both foods and herbs. This includes both their inherent potencies and how these can be altered through various preparations or combinations.[36] Once we learn to taste and imbibe the Shakti in foods and herbs, they gain a healing power far beyond their particular chemical constituents. They can also set in motion transformative processes in the mind and heart.

To work with the healing Shakti of plants, a good practice is to select one special healing herb and learn to work with its healing power as a power of the Goddess. Use that plant as one's Ishta Devata or chosen deity among the plants, as it were. Special plants used for this in India include aloe vera, holy basil (tulsi), turmeric, bael and neem, as well as the sacred banyan or Ashvattha tree. We can also use our local aromatics like sagebrush, mint, juniper or rose—in fact, any plant that we resonate with. Herbal teas convey the Shakti of the plant that has effects not only on the body but also the mind and nervous system.

Healing and Shakti

Shakti is the very force of healing, starting with the energy of awareness that brings balance and integration into all that it examines. Different healing therapies have their specific Shaktis, like the healing power of massage and therapeutic touch. Pranic or energy healing is also a kind of 'Shakti healing,' as it works directly through the cosmic energy. But it requires that the therapist resonates inwardly with the power of Shakti, which rests on wisdom, devotion and inner vitality.

For optimal healing, the appropriate healing Shakti needs to be applied relative to the particular imbalances within the person. This internal Shakti in Ayurvedic medicine is defined in terms of *Ojas*, or the immune strength, physical and emotional endurance, peace, balance and contentment of the person. People with good Ojas will live longer, have more mental stability and be spiritually more at peace. Their healing powers can be immense. To develop this Ojas or inner power, one must be able to hold one's Prana or life-force within, directing to the cosmic powers, not simply to outer worldly enjoyment. Ayurveda contains many special rejuvenation therapies to increase Ojas.[37]

The main Shakti or power of healing rests in Prana itself. It is the Prana, the vital energy from the food, herbs, massage and other treatment methods, which works to heal us. Different therapies are simply various means of creating and directing prana in different ways. Ultimately, it is the Prana of the healer that is the key factor or healing Shakti, and how that aligns with the Prana of the patient.

The best way to begin a healing process is through honoring of Shakti, both as a general life-force and in the specific therapies that may be employed. We should honor the healing Shakti both in the therapist and the patient, and seek its grace for the treatment to occur without obstruction.

A clinic or treatment room should be a temple to Shakti. Keeping special healing Shaktis present there aids in this process. This means that the treatment room or clinic should contain special plants, flowers, pleasant aromas, colors, gems, geometrical patterns, and other forms and symbols of the Goddess. Daily rituals, chanting, music, mantra and meditation should go on in order to create the sacred space of healing for the Shakti of healing to manifest. To honor the Goddess as the source of Shakti is even better.

Shakti and the Three Doshas

Ayurvedic medicine is based upon a recognition of three *doshas* or primary 'biological humors' of *Vata* (wind), *Pitta* (fire) and *Kapha* (water). These three are the prime factors behind both our biological functioning and the disease process. One of the doshas usually places its characteristic mark on the constitutional type of the person, as Vata (air) types, Pitta (fire) types, and Kapha (water types). Ayurvedic diets and life-style therapies are designed according to these.

We could say that the three doshas are the three main biological forms of Shakti. Each dosha is a powerful force at work throughout our anatomy and physiology. The three doshas in turn reflect deeper healing powers of *Prana* (Vata) or vital energy, *Tejas* (Pitta) or inner energy, and *Ojas* (Kapha) or underlying endurance. This primary Prana is the healing essence of air and life. Tejas is the healing essence of fire, light and heat. Ojas is the healing essence of water, emotion and nourishment.[38]

These three subtle forces in turn reflect the three great cosmic powers of *Vayu* (Prana) or the cosmic wind and lightning force, *Agni* (Tejas) or the cosmic fire, *Soma* (Kapha) or the cosmic waters, and the light powers of Lightning, Fire and Moon. They are reflected in three energy centers in the subtle body with the Moon and Soma relating to the crown chakra, Fire or Agni to the root chakra and Vayu or Wind to the heart chakra.

One can heal the doshas at a yogic level through accessing these three higher powers by way of pranayama (Wind), mantra (Fire) and meditation (the Moon). In this way, we can use our own internal Shaktis to change the energetics of both body and mind.

Learn to become receptive to the healing Shaktis of nature around you as the powers of your own inner nature and as your link with the Goddess or Divine Mother. All the healing powers in the universe belong to you, starting with Prana or life-energy that is the universal force. All healing Shaktis are powers of your own deeper Self, the grace that the Supreme Shakti has provided for your well-being on all levels. Learn to bring the Shakti of healing out of your deepest heart and unite it with the great reservoir of cosmic energy that pervades all of space, so that we can restore balance and harmony in the world around us.

PART THREE

The Forms and Personalities of the Goddess

*Seeing your special form subtle like a streak of Lightning,
made up of the Sun, Moon and Fire, placed above the six
chakras, great yogis with their minds purified from the impu-
rities of Maya, hold the perception of you in the thousand
petal lotus as the supreme wave of bliss,.*

SHANKARACHARYA, *SAUNDARYA LAHARI* 21

The following section examines several important Hindu Goddesses who
personify the universal Shakti, primarily Kali, Sundari and Bhairavi.
Through these personifications of the Divine feminine power, we can
communicate with the cosmic energy directly and gain its grace and support for all that we do.

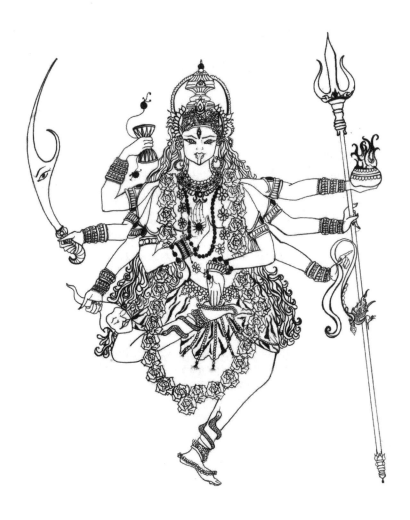

Nritya Kali

The Personality of Shakti

The universal Shakti or cosmic power, though it appears inanimate in its actions through the forces of nature, has its own personality. In fact, the Goddess has the most amazing and engaging personality because all energy, magic and beauty dwells within her. This 'Personality of the Goddess' has been honored and worshipped in spiritual traditions throughout the world and is arguably key to the most ancient and natural religion of humanity.

Of course, one may have a hard time investing the forces of nature with a personality, much less the grace and charisma of a Goddess! But as we observe the beauty and wonder of the universe around us, we can easily sense a Divine face behind it. Mother Nature is known to all of us, but perhaps we have not looked deeply enough into all that she is, which extends far beyond our earthly environment, to see the Goddess behind her.

The primal form of the Goddess is an ethereal form of lightning or electrical energy inherent in all existence. The electrical body of the Goddess pervades all of space and vibrates with all the sensory potentials through which we can experience life. It is the basis of not only the wonders of the galaxy but of the intricacies of our own minds and nervous systems!

127

Lightning has the speed, variability, beauty and delight of the feminine nature. To be able to see the personality of the Goddess inherent in lightning is to begin to approach the Goddess in her real majesty. The forces of nature are not mere physical formations working mechanically, but great Goddesses, expressions of a vaster life and consciousness. There is a feminine spirit, a beauty, frivolity and unpredictability in the wind, the water, the clouds, and the rain. The forces of nature reflect the moods of the Goddess as she parades her beauty and charm before the Cosmic Spirit through the rhythms of time.

Most of us do not see this dance of Divine Love hidden in the play of Nature and Spirit. However, those among us whose inner eye is open can find an endless delight in the interplay of these two primal forces, which can be called 'Shiva and Shakti', 'Radha and Krishna' or other forms of the God and the Goddess, the cosmic masculine and feminine powers. Enlightened Yogis find bliss dwelling alone in Nature, experiencing the entire universe in their own being.

Most of us are unaware of our non-embodied companions in the world, which we treat as having no real awareness or life of their own. We think that only embodied beings have any sort of consciousness, not realizing that consciousness pervades everything, even the inanimate realm. We fail to communicate with the wind, fire, stars or waters around us, alienating ourselves from our greater Self and cosmic community.

The forces of nature are formations of the Conscious Universe with their own purpose, drama and display, relative to which our human life is at best a reflection and at worst a shadow. Calling out to them expands the horizons of our souls and awakens us to our real place in the universe. Let us break down the barriers of communication that arise from the human ego, and embrace not only plants and animals, but very planets and stars as alive and aware, including the ground on which we stand!

When we fail to recognize the presence of the Goddess within and around us, we miss the real beauty and splendor of life. We fail to access the universal power from which alone our real energy needs can be fulfilled, which is our inner need for the energy of consciousness! While recognizing the energy of Shakti, let us not forget her marvelous personalities, the Devis that are her manifestations. Her face and voice are hidden in every leaf, flower, snowflake and star, extending to all of time, space and beyond.

When we learn to communicate with the great personalities of the Goddess, they can open up all the secrets of the universe to us, reflecting a power greater than any possible technology. We can relate to the transformative forces of nature as we would with our own mother. This is the best foundation on which to approach the Goddess, who is the Mother of all.

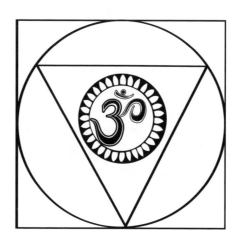

The Goddess Kali:
The Supreme Shakti of Infinite Space and Eternal Time

Kali is probably the most misunderstood and feared of all the great Hindu Goddesses. With her garland of skulls, head-chopper dripping blood, fangs, and dark body, her form is hard for many of us to look at. Kali has been given epithets like fierce, terrible, martial and cruel. She is associated with the powers of death and destruction.

This frightening appearance, however, is only the outer face of Kali, how she appears to those who are not awake in their inner minds and hearts, and even that is often portrayed in a crude manner. For those in whom the Yoga Shakti is awake, Kali is most beautiful, blissful and compassionate in appearance and in action. She is the universal form of the Goddess as Infinite Space, Eternal Time and Irresistible Energy. Her faces, eyes, ears and mind are everywhere. Her voice, arms and legs move and act on all planes of existence.

Kali is the power behind time and space that energizes everything through a secret electrical force. Without her sanction, not even a subatomic particle can stir for a microsecond. From her perspective, even the great clouds of galactic nebulae are but swirls of momentary dust settling at her lotus feet. It is this transcendent nature of Kali that makes her appear terrible to the outer vision, conditioned as we are to definable forms and forces within the boundaries of time, space and personality. Such a vision of Kali as terrible is not a true perception of her real nature. It is our ego reaction to her awesome power in which our human life becomes at best a reflection and at worst a falsehood. Though we may need to pass through the doorway of Kali's terror, it is only a movement of purification in order to discovery the blissful reality of Kali within all.

Kali is one of the many 'dark' forms of the Goddess, like the black Madonna. Her darkness is that of the earth, fertility, the night, boundless space, a cavern and the womb. It is a creative and transformative darkness, not one of limitation, ignorance or evil. It is the dark cloud from which both lightning and rain emerge, in order to produce life. The Dark Goddess is the form of mystery, secrecy, transition, origin and end. She represents the secret depth of all inner experience and spiritual realization.

Complementary to the dark forms of the Goddess are the white or light forms. Sarasvati, the Hindu Goddess of wisdom, is of this type, white in color, projecting pure virtue, grace and beauty in both her outer appearance and inner reality. The White Goddess and the Dark Goddess are not opposed to one another. They represent the alternating currents of day and night, creation and dissolution. Yet it is only when we face and transform the darkness—which is the action of Kali—that we can truly give birth to a light beyond desire, fear and duality.

The Meaning of Kali

The Sanskrit root 'kal', from which the name **Kālī** arises, has several meanings: 'to set and hold in motion' relative to time, 'to apportion and harmonize' relative to space, and 'to count' relative to form. At an inner level, it also means 'to think or to imagine', including 'to envision'. All these indications are relevant to the Goddess Kali.

Kali is the feminine form of time or **Kāla**. She is the Goddess of Time and Eternity, who is the silent witness of all things. Yet Kala does not just mean time in the abstract, Kala refers to the divisions of time, the rhythms of the days, months and seasons, through which the power of the Eternal and its recurrent waves of presence reveals itself. Kali is the Eternal energy that brings about all transformations in time of creation and destruction, birth and death.

Kali is also Infinite Space, not only as a background emptiness, but as the underlying matrix that allows things to hold their forms and sustain life. Her body is all of space, particularly its unmanifest realms beyond all creation, symbolized by her dark blue color.

Another important word deriving from the root 'kal', is **Kalā** meaning art, including music, dance, poetry and drama, which refers to the harmonious distribution of form, like the facets of a jewel. Kali is the embodiment of all the sixty-four arts and is also the power to give beauty for forms. A related term *Kalyani* also means beautiful and auspicious.

Kali has many different forms and manifestations; some which can be frightful. She is *Smashana Kali*, 'Kali who dwells in the cremation ground'. But her presence at death occurs to carry the soul out of the body and into the higher worlds. Kali is our savioress at the time of death, not the sorrow inherent in the process of dying. If we surrender to her grace, death becomes a transformation and liberation for the soul.

She is *Guhya Kali* or 'mysterious Kali', the energy that is hidden in secret places, in the womb, the cave, the night, the ground or the field of infinite space beyond the stars. Once we accept the energy of her paradox and ambiguity into our lives, which is the Self-existent mystery of all that is or ever can be, then our lives become magical and sublime, filled with subtle meanings in all that we experience.

She is *Bhadra Kali* or 'auspicious Kali'. Though Bhadra Kali is often depicted in a fierce form, her name suggests a kinder energy. By taking control over the powers of suffering, death and destruction,

Kali transforms them into tools of inner growth. She does not wield any negative power against her devotees, but removes all negativity from them for their benefit, which is the greatest of all blessings.

She is *Dakshina Kali* or 'Kali who has discrimination'. In this regard, Kali reflects *Dakshinamurti*, the youthful form of Shiva as the great world teacher who, seated under a banyan tree, can enlighten the most elderly rishis and yogis by the power of his silence alone. Kali has the enduring insight born of eternity, which makes her timeless and ever young. One need not strive to discriminate between the eternal and the transient in her presence. She infuses us with the eternal in which the transient does not simply fade away, but reveals itself as but a wave on the unending sea.

Kali does not simply negate the world into nothingness; she reveals the poignancy of the eternal presence mirrored in every transient event. Under her grace each experience gains a lasting significance, even simple daily activities like washing dishes or tending a garden. Through her vitalizing vision, the world becomes more wonderful, all of Nature becomes alive with the bliss currents of the supreme Brahman, and all the knots of sorrow in the heart are released into joy.

The fierce form of Kali destroys all the demons that assail us, the negative forces of ego and the turbulent emotions that pull us down in life. She conquers death itself, winning the greatest of all battles, that of the soul for immortal life. Kali represents the supreme victory of the Divine over all that is undivine, of light over darkness, truth over falsehood, the unlimited over the limited. Kali affords us the ecstasy of the greatest cosmic triumph, in which all suffering, pain and negativity are overcome forever in the Absolute. With her victory, all strife comes to an end for all time. Those who have surrendered to Kali can never die. For them, death is no enemy but simply a reflection of her deathless light.

However, to find the most blissful form of Kali, we must first be willing to let go of our own suffering, attachments, fears and desires. Notice I did not say that we must try to eliminate these things. We cannot and need not eliminate anything that is part of life. But we can release all things back into their origin in the Infinite and Eternal, like a stream flowing back into the sea. Once we stop holding on to things, every event in life will reveal itself into a Divine play and communicate to us a message of delight.

The Energy of Kali

The force of Kali is the most powerful energy that can direct us on our inner journey. She transforms the darkness into light, revealing the deeper spiritual radiance that is hidden behind all apparent obscurity. We need not fear her power but we cannot discover her grace unless we are willing to face our own fears, much like how a climber must challenge his fears in order to scale a high summit. Life is an adventure and its difficulties are the steep slopes that we encounter along the way. Let us not be overcome by such short term obstacles but be willing to make a greater effort to find the truth that is universal. Kali will be present at our side to provide the additional energy and skill, if we sincerely call upon her!

Out of the womb of Kali arises her lightning of Infinite Space and Eternal Time which keeps the entire universe in motion. Inwardly, her lightning power of perception awakens us to our own infinite and eternal nature. Her lightning prana invigorates us with eternal life, opening all the chakras and nadis within us. Her liquid lightning flows through the Yogi in currents of bliss, taking one beyond body and mind. Kali is the supreme *Yogini* or high priestess of Yoga, who guides our inner practice at every step from our initial disappointment with ordinary life to our final merging in the supreme Brahman.

From the standpoint of the inner awareness, eternal time becomes infinite space. Instead of a movement from past to future, time becomes like space, an endless expanse with neither beginning nor end. One can move to different places in time just as one might move to different locations in space, grasping all time as a single moment. This type of 'time travel', in which one goes beyond time, is one of the transcendent visions of Kali, who breaks down all the divisions of time and space.

The Eternal and the Infinite are one in an endless presence and can be grasped in a single moment and in a single point, as a pure focus. It is out of this universal focus that Kali's lightning arises. Kali smiles on us from within and beyond all things, as the center and the horizon of all possibilities.

Kali is not only eternity as beyond time, she is the dynamic power within time to transform all things. She divides eternity into the phases and rhythms of time, which constitute her endless dance. She reflects the beauty of eternity into the movements of time through the day, month, year, life time and world age up to the very life of the entire universe. All the movements of time are but waves on the sea of eternity. They are Kali's play as she weaves eternity into ever new forms and expressions, through the light of the heavenly bodies that she sets in motion by her grace.

Kali is not only Infinite Space but the power of place and direction within space. Each location in space is formation of the geography of the Infinite. Each place has its own Shakti, which is its unique power to express some aspect of infinity in a special way. This 'power of the place' is reflected in the geology and geography of the place and the action of the creatures within it. In this regard, we can find the infinite and unlimited in every place. Each place that we visit has something new to show us, something that we have not seen before, which can function for us as a window to the infinite.

Each direction of space brings us some portion of the Infinite energy, from spiritual power in the northeast, the direction of *Ishana*, the Divine force of inspiration, to worldly submission in the southwest, the direction of *Nirriti*, the worldly force of control and destruction, as clearly explained in *Vastu Shastra*, the Vedic directional science. All directions are facets of the spatial power of Kali to create life and change. Kali is the circle whose center is everywhere and circumference is nowhere, yet her curves give shape to everything and provide the impetus for everything to return back to her again.

As the eternal and the infinite interpenetrate, so do Kali's powers of time and place. Time as our experience gives power to a place, making it meaningful for us. Similarly, the place where we live lends power to time and makes the events experienced there more meaningful for us. These are all the gifts of the great Goddess. When we see her power and her beauty in all times and all places, then we transcend time and space, and become one with Kali, from the silence and stillness of the Supreme Shiva, with which she is ever united.

Kali as the Yoga Shakti

Kali is the primary Goddess of Yoga, the background *Yoga Shakti*, the power of yogic action or Kriya. She reflects inner magnetism that draws our energy within, which causes us to seek the eternal and lose interest in the outer affairs of life. Kali is the electrical stirring of the soul to Divinity. She is the Divine voice reverberating within us with great transformative force. She is the Divine will working through us with an indomitable impetus, which arises when we let our little self fade into the background.

Kali is the great Prana or cosmic life-force that is the life blood of the universe. She represents the most primal desire of all living beings, the wish to live forever and to never die. This core longing for immortality is not some mere delusion or arrogance; it is the very reflection of *Sat* or 'Pure Being' into creation, the portion of the Eternal that constitutes our soul.

Kali also represents the primal power of Divine love, which is to find the perfect, pure and eternal union, the presence of Shiva, the Eternal Being and Consciousness hidden in all life. Behind even our ordinary desires is Kali's ascending force stirring us to seek something more beautiful and wondrous, to make us unhappy with what we have accumulated, in order to move us towards a greater reality beyond, until we go beyond the entire universe to the endless fields of the Absolute.

Kali's will generates the decisive moment of spiritual awakening within us, in which we realize that true happiness cannot be found in the outer world but only within. Then she reorients our life as a mystic journey to the inner source, the heart of creation, the Eternal flame. We are reborn as a Divine soul, conscious of its many births and of its eventual goal to go beyond all time to its Eternal abode.

Kali's Shakti enables us to focus our energies within, to take them back to the heart and core of our being. Kali's inner process is to reverse the order of creation and return us to the Absolute. Hers is the power that merges earth into water, water into fire, fire into air, air into ether, ether into mind, and mind into pure consciousness. She takes us back from the many to the One, reintegrating the world into our deepest Self.

This means that Kali's energy is like a simulated death experience. She helps us withdraw our attention from the outer mind, emotions and senses into the inner heart. In this regard, Kali is the prime Goddess of *Jnana* or Self-knowledge. She merges us back into the Self in the heart, unifying all our experience within our deepest feeling and knowing. Kali is *Nirvana Shakti*, the power that takes us to dissolution or Nirvana. She is the magnetic pull of Nirvana within us.

In Yogic terms, Kali is the *Nirodha Shakti*, the power that dissolves the fluctuations of the mind or chitta. Her power checks, negates, masters and dissolves all the agitations of mind and prana into the infinite silent calm of the Purusha within the heart. Not surprisingly, Kali is the main Goddess worshipped by great yogis.

One is reminded of the experience of Ramakrishna, who was a great devotee of Kali. After learning the Self-knowledge of Vedanta through his guru Tota Puri, Ramakrishna meditated on the

Self within the heart in order to realize it. In doing so, the image of Kali arose instead. He learned that he had to break through his attachment to her by removing her form with the sword of knowledge. Yet he eventually came to realize that the sword of knowledge was also the sword of Kali. Kali projects a form, an appearance of the Goddess, to guide us along the way, but dissolves her form when it has fulfilled its purpose, which is to bring us back to the eternal state of peace and equipoise within her formless Being.

Kali and Her Mantras

Each deity or Devata has its mantras, which reflect its energies, names and forms of knowledge that serve to awaken the deity within us. These mantras start with a single-syllable seed or bija mantras and extend to longer mantras, prayers and supplications. They may be recited as part of external rituals, pranayama, and meditation or by themselves. Such mantras are the main yogic tool to work with the deity and its powers.

Kali's Bija Krīm

Kali's primary single syllable mantra is **Krīm**. **Krīm** refers to Kriya or the power of action, but action of a yogic nature. **Krīm** is composed of three primary letters.

- The letter–**ka** is the first consonant in the Sanskrit alphabet. It indicates manifest existence, power and force, including time, place and action.
- The letter–**ra** is the seed sound of the fire element and light, both outwardly and inwardly.
- The letter–ī indicates focused energy, motivation and will power, Shakti as an executive force.

Krīm as the sound of Kali is the primary force of life, creation and manifestation. It is the original energy or lightning that sets everything in motion, like an electric current. When we use this mantra in our Yoga practice, we are switching on the inner current of Shakti. Through it we can empower any practice or awaken any inner faculty, just like having the electricity on in our house that can be used to run various appliances.

The great Goddess Kali, through her mantra **Krīm**, provides us the support energy for all that we attempt in Yoga. She increases our inner strength and endurance, both allowing and pushing us to do more. Her mantra creates a relentless force of spiritual energy within us that propels and guides us to the higher goal. At some point her current takes over and directs our practice by its flow, with our own will surrendered to her. This opens up a higher level of practice beyond the personal, with the Divine Shakti directing our inner growth.

The mantra **Krīm** has a fierce side and like a jolt of lightning or like a sword can cut things open. It can stimulate, shock, electrify or propel. It can energize the weapons of the Gods to defeat the undivine or Asuric forces. Yet it can also energize the ornaments of the Gods, their gems and gifts, which grant bliss to the devotee. If you want to practice this mantra, remember it is a strong mantra that should be approached after one has already first used **Hrīm**, the benefic mantra of the Goddess, to connect with her grace in your heart.

Kali's Threefold Bija: Krīm Hūm Hrīm

Out of this single seed mantra is developed a longer threefold mantra or three seed-mantras as **Krīm Hūm Hrīm**. This threefold mantra has more energy and efficacy in awakening the Goddess within us. It begins with the mantra **Krīm** and builds upon its power.

The mantra **Hūm** is composed of two primary sounds. The letter-**ha** is the seed syllable of the element of space or ether. It also represents the Sun, Prana and the Purusha principle of pure consciousness. The letter-**ū** creates a force field that can both serve to hold positive energy in and to push negative energy out. **Hūm** represents an explosion of energy, an expression of great power that is pranic, electrical and fiery. **Hūm** is the power of Agni or fire, particularly as directed by the wind or Vayu. Whereas **Krīm** awakens the electrical force or Shakti, **Hūm** serves to direct it with great force and to use it to make great efforts.

Hrīm is the great mantra of the spiritual heart, *hridaya*. It is composed of three main letters. The letter-**Ha**, as in **Hūm**, represents, space, prana and light. The letter-**Ra** as in **Krīm** represents light and fire. The letter-**Ī** as in **Krīm** represents focused energy or a ray of light, the Shakti as such. Through the mantra **Hrīm** alone, one can enter into the spiritual heart and the small space within its lotus in which the entire universe is held.[39]

These put together, Kali's threefold mantra serves to awaken and energize the spiritual heart.

- The mantra **Krīm** serves to cut the knots of the heart. It works like a sword. It stimulates the heart energy within us, its primal desire or wish for immortality, love and light.
- The mantra **Hūm** gives power to the heart, expanding the energy of prana and Agni (fire) in a strong, if not explosive manner.
- The mantra **Hrīm** opens the energy of the spiritual heart which is like the Sun, spreading it into the Infinite.

This threefold Kali Heart mantra can be compared to a kind of spiritual adrenaline. **Krīm** awakens the energy of the heart, like an electrical jolt to a heart patient whose heart is failing. **Hūm** expands it this current with great force. **Hrīm** stabilizes it as an infinite power and eternal presence.

Krīm draws the Prana from the breath, the sensory and motor organs and directs it into the heart. **Hūm** turns the Prana into a force of fiery meditative power. Hrīm connects the individual prana-mind with the power of the Supreme Self, the power of the light of consciousness (Chid-jyoti). This threefold mantra there-fore creates a powerful pratyahara in the yogic sense; it takes our energy back to the spiritual heart.

When we place these three mantras in another order as Hrīm Krīm Hūm, they become a weapon and can be used to remove neg-ativities from the body and mind. This directs the Supreme Shakti from the inner heart to dissolve all that opposes the higher truth.

Kali's Sevenfold Mantra

Kali's sevenfold mantra is an extension of the threefold mantra, repeating Krīm three times and Hūm and Hrīm two times each. This emphasizes the power of Krīm.

Krīm Krīm Krīm Hūm Hūm Hrīm Hrīm

After having energized the threefold Kali mantra, you can go on to this sevenfold mantra, repeating it while meditating upon Kali and seeking her grace. You can repeat this mantra once upon inhala-tion, once upon retention and once upon exhalation. In this way it will begin to energize your prana at a higher level, aligning it with the transcendent Prana of Kali.

Kali's Extended Mantra

Kali has a longer or extended mantra that does not only repeat her bija mantras, but calls to her by name. It repeats her sevenfold mantra twice, invoking her in between as Dakshina Kali, and end-ing with Svaha, the fire offering mantra.

Krīm Krīm Krīm Hūm Hūm Hrīm Hrīm, Dakṣine Kālike,
Krīm Krīm Krīm Hūm Hūm Hrīm Hrīm, Svāhā!

This mantra is specific for her knowledge or Dakshina form. Invoking Kali by name adds greater power and efficacy to the mantra and calls her to us. In this great mantra Kali functions as a kind of 'spiritual adrenaline' to awaken the spiritual heart, which for most of us is inert, slumbering or not functioning at all. Those who repeat it find a tremendous and irresistible power carrying them forward on their inner path. But it is only for those who have the devotion to Kali and who approach it with inner calm and determination.

Kali Sadhana and the Yoga of Knowledge

Kali mantras serve to develop a *Kali Sadhana*, the 'Inner Yoga of Kali', in which the true nature of Kali is revealed. Kali is the death of the ego, which is the spiritual rebirth or resurrection of the soul. Kali is the Divine Mother in her role of slaying the demon or dragon of the ego and giving birth to the Divine Child of Self-awareness within us. Her mantras bring about an inner death, which is the rebirth of the immortal Self within us.

Through Kali we can experience a simulated death, a complete forgetting of this outer world for the inner reality. Kali takes us through the real death, which is that of the ego, after which there is no more death for the soul. Kali is this 'death of death' by the power of eternity. She represents the complete victory of the powers of knowledge, light and truth over the forces of ignorance, darkness and falsehood. Hers is the greatest accomplishment; the end of all negativity, limitation and sorrow, even in the midst of what outwardly may appear as death, pain and suffering.

Kali mantras are a powerful means to move into the spiritual heart, the seat of the inner light and life. They are a good accompaniment to the practice of 'Self-inquiry', the meditation on the Great Question 'Who am I?' and related approaches of the Yoga of Knowledge.[40]

The Goddess Kali is the power of meditation personified as a Goddess. Kali is the natural state of meditation as the power of consciousness pervading Infinite Space and Eternal Time, in which the waves of karma, birth and death, cannot touch us. Kali's mantras take us to the highest knowledge. They are not just devotional expressions but the very energy of the Absolute absorbing its own creation in ecstasy and joy.

Kali and the Power of the Sacrifice

All Tantric and Vedic deities represent various ways of sacrifice or manifestations of the sacred. Yoga itself is an inner sacrifice of speech, breath and mind into the indwelling deity, the Divine Self within the heart.[41] Tantric deities are deeply rooted in the older Vedic sacrifice—the Vedic sense of all life as a sacrificial offering to the Divine through the sacred fire—not only in an historical sense but as part of the same understanding of life and consciousness.

The Goddess Kali is first mentioned in the ancient *Upanishads* as the first of the seven tongues of Agni or the sacred fire, which are conceived of all feminine in nature in the *Vedas*.[42] She is the tongue of the sacred fire that consumes all the offerings. In Tantra, Kali also relates to the tongue of the Goddess. Since the Goddess is first of all the power of speech, the tongue can be regarded as her supreme power. Note that Kali's Yantra or geometrical form when represented with an upward pointing triangle symbolizes the tongue and her power of speech. When her Yantra uses a downward pointing triangle it represents her power of creation through the womb.

The Goddess Durga is first mentioned in the *Upanishads* as arising from the Soma offering to Agni, the sacred fire, as *Jatavedas*, the

145

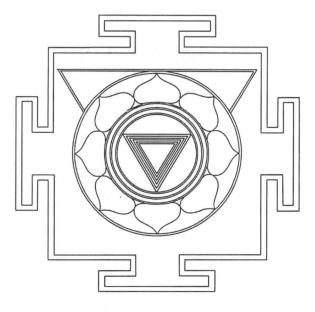

KALI YANTRA

Knower of all births, in order to protect us from our enemies. [43] In the Vedic *Sri Sukta*, which is the first hymn to the Goddess Lakshmi, it is Agni as Jatavedas who conveys the Goddess to us.[44] Therefore, it is important to be aware of the Vedic symbolism behind Tantric Goddesses, including their fierce forms, whose weapons and gestures have their reflection in the sacrificial process.

All Hindu deities have two main aspects as 'benefic', *Saumya* (watery, soft or Soma-related), or 'malefic', *Agneya* (fiery, harsh or Agni related). This is true of Shiva who is both fierce as Rudra, Ugra or Bhairava and kind as Shiva, Shankara, Shambhu and Soma. It is true of the Devi who is both fierce as Kali, Chandi and Bhairavi and soft as Lakshmi, Kamala, Lalita, and Sundari. These two sides of the deities reflect the Soma and Agni aspects of the sacrifice, as the power of the sacrifice to burn and purify (Agni) or to grant blessings and rain (Soma).

Vedic sacrifices or *Yajnas* are not simply rituals to be performed by human beings but reflect prime cosmic processes and events. Everything in the universe is a sacrificial interaction as it were, receiving and giving, taking in and letting out. Everything we do on a biological level is a kind of sacrifice. Eating is the first of the bodily Yajnas, an offering of food to the digestive fire (Jatharagni). Breathing is an offering of the inhaled air to the Pranic fire (Pranagni). Sensation is offering sensory impressions into the fire of the mind (Manasika Agni). Yajna is not simply sacrifice in the crude or outer sense, but the way of transformation inherent in the movement of life, in which all things are interrelated.

All cosmic processes are Yajnas or transformative actions. The very movement of time is the greatest Yajna or sacrificial offering of life, comprising creation and destruction, birth and death of all creatures and all worlds. The cosmic form of Agni in the *Vedas* called *Vaishvanara*, or the 'Universal Person', indicates the supreme power of time. The same deity is referred to as *Kalagni Rudra*, Rudra as the fire of time, the fierce form of Shiva, whose powerful cosmic dance or *Tandava*, dissolves the universe into Divine fire and light.

Kali Yajna

The great Goddess Kali personifies the power of the *Kala Yajna*, the 'Time Sacrifice' or sacrificial movement of time. Everything born is a time sacrifice, an offering into the fire of eternity. Everything that arises through birth must be offered back to the womb of time through the process of death. Our entire lives in the field of time consist of taking and giving, partaking of the communion of all that is.

Kali's fierce appearance—holding a cut off head and wearing a garland of skulls—symbolizes the Kala Yajna in which creatures are born, grow, mature, decay and die. Kali herself represents the force of spiritual growth, the ongoing development of the soul that occurs in the life process. The garland of skulls represents the collection of past lives of the soul. The cut off head indicates the ego unaware of the process of rebirth, blinding thinking it is the true being and its particularly life is the only one. Kali as the time sacrifice teaches us to be aware of our soul's work in life and the need to develop it through yogic practices.

Kali as space is the 'Space Sacrifice' or *Akasha Yajna*. All objects in the universe are combinations of the five great elements of earth, water, fire, air and ether, which all develop from and return to the womb of space. Everything that exists is a flower arising from space and eventually returns to space. Space pervades and surrounds us on every side without and within. Life can only exist in the body because of the space, cavities and channels within it. The mind can only perceive and think because of its ability to reflect things through space. Kali is the great matrix of space, of which all forms are but waves, a dance or a dream.

Kali as Prana, the cosmic life force, is the *Prana Yajna*, the 'Life Sacrifice', which is indicated through our biological processes, particularly eating and breathing. Kali is the cosmic Prana that is the eater of everything in the universe. The entire universe is food for or a feast for the soul.

Kali is the cosmic breath that breathes through all creatures. All breaths are really hers and are sustained only by her power. Kali is the cosmic blood that energizes the flow of blood in all creatures. All blood belongs to her, and as the great Prana, she is ever drinking the blood of everyone. This is the mystic meaning why Kali is portrayed with blood on her tongue.

Kali is the *Karma Yajna*, the 'karma sacrifice' that is the process of action and its consequences. Karma itself in Sanskrit refers to a Yajna, a ritual, and does not just indicate ordinary action. Action that serves to create strong karmas is action that is energized by thought, intention, desire and will-power and is performed regularly, cyclically and repeatedly. It thereby also becomes a ritual.

Karma in the ordinary sense of action is a Yajna or sacrifice, starting with our biological rituals of sleeping, bathing, eating and exercising. Our actions are a Yajna in which we are offering ourselves to the forces of the universe. The problem is that we forget we are performing a Yajna and so act in an unsacred manner that leads us to corruption and suffering. We exploit the sacred universe for our own egoistic ends, forgetting the greater sacrificial urge of the soul and its need to grow in consciousness through recognizing and honoring the sacred everywhere.

Kali personifies the great truths of the sacrifice. She is not a terrible Goddess but a magnificent portrayal of cosmic reality in powerful symbolic terms. She herself is the sacrificed Goddess, particularly in the related form of *Sati*, who offers her own body up in the sacred fire, or as *Chinnamasta*, who cuts her own head off. In this regard, Kali is akin to sacrificed male Gods and saviors like Osiris, Adonis, and Jesus. While we may find her symbolism harder to understand, if we look deeply it is pointing at the same inner truth.

The syllable **Ka** also indicates desire, which is the basis of all life. The syllable **Li** indicates *laya* or 'mergence'. Kali is both the summit and the end of all desires. This is the movement of the sacrifice. To worship Kali means to see everything as a Divine sacrifice, the Godhead offering itself in manifestation for the evolution of consciousness. Kali is the power of the sacrifice to bring about great transformations, to call down the flow of heavenly grace or Soma, to make sure that we make the real, complete and decisive offering that takes us beyond the realm of limitation.

We cannot truly practice Yoga unless we view it as an inner sacrifice or self-offering to the Divine. Otherwise the asanas, pranayamas, mantras and meditations we do remain limited to the ordinary human sphere. True Yoga begins with selfless sacrifice as

Karma Yoga, which is action done in recognition and honor of the sacred. The great powers or Devatas of Yoga are the powers of sacrifice. They function for the sanctification or making sacred of all things in life, from our blood and bones, to the rivers and mountains, to our breath and thought.

To discover the sacred nature of reality, our lives must become an inner offering to the Divine, a yogic sacrifice. By honoring all things as sacred we can discover the sacred eternal presence that is Brahman, the Absolute beyond all time, space and action. Deity Yoga helps return us to the Sacred Reality that is the essence of all the Gods and Goddesses. Kali is a personification of the sacrifice to lead us to the sacred within and beyond all things, to the highest Reality.

The Goddess Sundari
and the Flow of Soma

The dominant form of the Goddess worshiped in South India and its great Tantric traditions is *Tripura Sundari,* the 'Beauty of the Three Worlds' or *Sundari* or the 'Beautiful One'. Sundari is a deity of bliss, union and delight. She is aligned with other benefic forms of the Goddess like *Lalita,* 'She Who Plays', *Rajarajeshvari,* 'The Supreme Queen of the Universe', *Matangi,* 'Whose Mind is full of passion,' and *Bhuvaneshvari,* 'The Queen of the World'.

At an esoteric level, Sundari is the key deity for the practice of Sri Vidya and the worship of the Sri Chakra, the highest of all Tantric teachings. *Her fifteenfold mantra called the 'Panchadashi' is regarded as the most powerful and important of all Tantric mantras. It is the Tantric equivalent of the Gayatri mantra, the most important of the Vedic mantras.*

The Goddess Tripura Sundari is the main deity governing the flow of *Soma,* mystic nectar or *amrit,* from the crown chakra. She opens the thousand petals of the crown chakra and releases their thousand currents of Soma which flood the body and mind with bliss. She relates to the mind, *manas* in Sanskrit, in the deepest sense as the power of pure contemplation.

151

Sundari is the inner power of the mind that grants us the knowledge of all mantras, the thousand syllables, through which all wisdom comes to us as a delight to the soul. There are more great hymns of praise to Sundari in Sanskrit literature than to any other Goddess, including some of the most beautiful works in the language, as she is the very font of poetic inspiration.

Sundari is the full Moon dispensing its attractive and delightful luminosity on all the worlds, as the Moon is the crown chakra in yogic thought. Yet she is not merely the Moon as a heavenly body but the cooling blissful energy inherent in the light of consciousness, which does not burn us but fills us with delight. The highest spiritual light has a cooling effect upon the mind, ushering in love and peace, which is the light of Sundari and Soma.

Sundari is the bliss of Brahman (Brahmananda) and provides the realization that that 'the entire universe is Brahman', *Sarvam Khalvidam Brahma.* In this regard, she is an important deity of Advaita or non-dualistic Vedanta and the Yoga of Knowledge. She is lauded by the great Advaitic guru Shankaracharya in his most famous poem, and indeed, the most famous of all Tantric poems to the Goddess, *Saundarya Lahari,* 'the Wave of Beauty'.

Sundari is both opposite and complementary in nature to Kali. She is the light form of the Goddess relative to Kali's dark form, the beauty to Kali's terror. She is the supreme white Goddess, as it were, to balance Kali as the black Goddess. Sundari balances the dynamic power of Kali, which is dominated by the fire and air elements, with her soothing watery flow. She is the magnetic counterpart of Kali's surging electrical energy.

By meditating upon both Kali and Sundari, one takes one's energies to a higher level, avoiding any fixation on negativity through an exclusive worship of Kali, or attachment to beautiful forms through an exclusive worship of Sundari. It is best to balance both Kali and Sundari for a harmonious and integral practice.

Sundari's Mantras

Sundari's Single Bija

Sundari's single or bija mantra is the sound **Klīm**. Klīm is the *Kama bija* or seed syllable of desire, love, imagination, deep feeling and attachment. It grants the fulfillment of all the real wishes of the heart, the true desires of the soul.[45] Whatever it is that we truly desire in our hearts, not merely the wants of the ego, can be fulfilled by the repetition of this mantra and a deep devotion to the Goddess. As this is a benefic mantra, one can freely repeat it to increase love and devotion.

Sundari's Threefold Mantra

Sundari's three syllable mantra is **Aim Klīm Sauḥ**. This mantra is specific to her *Shodashi* or *Bala* form, her aspect as a sixteen year old girl. It is one of the most powerful of all the threefold mantras. It develops out of the bija **Klīm** and expands its power to grant all wishes. This extraordinary mantra is said to be able to rejuvenate the mind and the nervous system, to counter stress, anxiety, pain and grief.[46] It has the same power as the longer Panchadashi mantra, but is easier to recite.

Aim is the mantra of Adi Shakti, the Supreme Shakti, being to the Goddess what **OM** (**Aum**) is to Shiva. As **Aum** is the light of the mystic Sun, **Aim** is the light of the mystic Moon. **Aum** is the supreme Purusha or Shiva. **Aim** is the supreme Devi or Shakti. **Aim** is pure existence (**A**) plus Shakti or the Goddess (**I**). **Aum** is pure existence (**A**) plus Ishvara or the Cosmic Lord (**U**).

On a more specific level, the mantra **Aim** relates to the power of the Divine Word, inspired speech, poetic ability and mantra in general. That is why it is connected to the Goddess Sarasvati, the Goddess of Wisdom, and to the guru. Chant **Aim** as you think of the guru and you can contact him at a telepathic level.

Sauḥ allows for the flow of Soma and the dispensation of the light of the Moon. It is the mantra of Shakti in expression, as an effusion of the heart. It takes the prime vowel sound -**Au** as in **Aum**, which carries the power of consciousness. To this it adds the consonant-**S**, which gives Shakti, stability, purity and prana. The final-**H**, sound, a half-**Ha** called *Visarga* in Sanskrit, serves to project the energy, allowing the Soma to descend from the crown chakra to the heart and the entire body.

Sundari's Fivefold Mantra
Sundari has a five syllable mantra—**Hrīm Śrīm Klīm Aim Sauḥ**—which is also quite transformative. It begins with the mantra of the heart **Hrīm**, followed by the mantra of devotion **Śrīm** and then the mantra of Divine Love and Desire, **Klīm**. This is followed by **Aim**, which is the primal Shakti of speech and **Sauḥ**, which causes the grace of the previous four mantras to flow.

This is a very benefic mantra which calms the heart and the nervous system and grants the fulfillment of our deeper desires. It is an expansion of the threefold mantra **Aim Klīm Sauḥ**, which it contains.

Sundari's Supreme Fifteenfold Mantra: the Panchadashi Mantra
Sundari's longer or extended mantra is the famous Panchadashi or fifteen syllable mantra. It is the primary mantra behind the geometrical form of the Sri Chakra, the most powerful and elaborate of all the yantras. It is said to be the most powerful of all Tantric mantras, spiritualizing speech, prana and mind.

Ka E Ī La Hrīm, Ha Sa Ka Ha La Hrīm, Sa Ka La Hrīm

There also is a 'sixteenfold' or *Shodashi* version of the mantra, which can be formed in two different manners. The first is to add the mantra **Śrīm** to the end of the Panchadashi mantra, which brings more calm to the mind and heart, consecrating the mantra through devotion and surrender:

Ka E Ī La Hrīm, Ha Sa Ka Ha La Hrīm, Sa Ka La Hrīm Śrīm

The second is to begin the mantra with another **Hrīm**. In this way the entire mantra becomes a protracted **Hrīm** or laudation of the Goddess in the spiritual heart.

Hrīm Ka E Ī La Hrīm, Ha Sa Ka Ha La Hrīm, Sa Ka La Hrīm

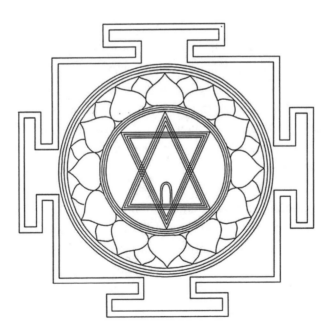

TRIPURA SUNDARI YANTRA

There is also a *Purna* or 'complete' form of the mantra, adding
aspects of the fivefold Sundari mantra to it. It works quite well
and is very intoxicating.

Śrīm Hrīm Klīm Aim Sauḥ, Om Hrīm Śrīm, Ka E I La Hrīm, Ha
Sa Ka Ha La Hrīm, Sa Ka La Hrīm, Sauḥ Aim Klīm Hrīm Śrīm

Yet another form is to add the threefold Bala Sundari mantra
to it (**Aim Klīm Sauḥ**), one syllable for each section with **Aim** as
the power of speech, **Klīm** as the power of Prana, and **Sauḥ** as the
energy of the mind.

Aim Ka E Ī La Hrīm, Klīm Ha Sa Ka Ha La Hrīm,
Sauḥ Sa Ka La Hrīm

There are many other variations on this magical mantra, either in terms of the syllables which compose it or those that can
be added to it. Well over a hundred such variations can be found
in Tantric lore, relating to various deities and rishis. One should
only take up this mantra after having repeated the other shorter
Sundari mantras. But do so with caution, attention and devotion
to the Goddess.

Explanation of the Panchadashi Mantra
The Panchadashi mantra, like the Sri Yantra, contains the entire
universe and our entire nature, from the physical to the Absolute
or Supreme Brahman. It holds the greatest and most secret of all
yogic teachings in a cryptic mantric language which, from a few
syllables can unfold and expand to encompass all of existence.

The mantra comes in three sections:

The first section (**Ka E Ī La Hrīm**) relates to Vak or the power
of speech and is called *Vagkuta* or the 'pinnacle of speech'. It corresponds to the region of Fire or Agni and the three lower chakras,

the root, sex and navel, which is awakened through the power of speech. It unfolds the feminine aspect of speech as the Goddess.

The second section (**Ha Sa Ka Ha La Hrīm**) relates to Prana and is called *Kamaraja* or the 'King of all desires'. It corresponds to the region of the Sun or Surya and the three middle chakras, the navel, heart and throat, specifically the heart. It contains Pranic sounds like s-sounds and h-sounds that energize the heart. It energizes the feminine aspect of Prana as the Goddess.

The third section (**Sa Ka La Hrīm**) relates to the Mind and is called *Shaktikuta* or the 'pinnacle of Shakti'. It corresponds to the region of the Moon or Soma, the higher three chakras of the throat, third eye and head, specifically the head or crown chakra. It energizes the feminine aspect of the mind as the Goddess.

This fifteenfold mantra repeats several key sounds. The great mantra of the Goddess, **Hrīm**, is repeated three times, once for each section, connecting each with the Supreme Shakti. **Hrīm** awakens the Kundalini Shakti and its power of Prana, Agni, light, space, power and delight. The third section mantra 'Sakala Hrīm' also means that everything (sakala) is **Hrīm**, which is light, beauty and delight. So the fifteen syllables of the mantra are really just extensions or glorifications of the mantra **Hrīm**, the Devi's most sacred sound.

The letters **Ka** and **La** appear in each of the three sections. Together they make the term 'kala' meaning a division, referring to the sixteen digits or phases (kalas) of the Moon. These sixteen aspects relate to the *Vishuddha* or throat chakra which has sixteen petals. Yet they relate to the thousand petal lotus of the head as well. They refer to all the divisions of energies in the universe, and ultimately all the powers of art called Kala.

Ka is the first of all consonants, as the letter-**A** is the first of all vowels in the Sanskrit alphabet. The letter-**A** represents unmanifest existence, pure being or the Absolute. In a similar way, the latter **Ka** represents manifest existence, life, identity, time, place, air, fire, karma, action and desire—that which sets everything in motion in the universe.

La is the seed sound for the earth element in Tantra and as such represents the limit, end or culmination of manifest existence and the creative urge, the fulfillment of desire or bliss. **Ka** and **La** as two sounds, therefore, contain the entire universe between them and represent the laws, rhythms and patterns of Shakti which sustains it.

The letters **Ha** and **Sa** both occur twice among the fifteen letters of this mantra. **Ha** and **Sa** are complementary sounds. **Ha** is exhalation or the expression of Prana, which stimulates speech and the motor organs. **Sa** is inhalation or the absorption of Prana, which feeds the cognitive senses and the mind. At a general level, **Ha** indicates Prana and **Sa** indicates the mind.

Ha occurs twice in the second or Pranic section of the mantra. **Ha** is the sound of the Sun, space and Prana, which this section of the mantra reflects as relating to Prana. **Sa** occurs once in each of the second and third sections of the mantra. Relating to the Moon, the mind and Shakti, the letter **Sa** has its unique place, beginning the third section of the mantra.

The first section of the mantra has two vowels, **E** and **I**, repeated only once. **E** is said to be the yoni or the womb of all manifestation. It is a diminutive form of the mantra **Aim**, or the seed of **Aim**, which represents the Divine Word or speech as the ruling and directing cosmic power. The letter-**E** holds all sounds latent within itself as the basis for their manifestation in later letters.

The letter **Ī**, pronounced 'ee', represents Shakti in general as will power, ruling power, executive force, design, motivation and electrical force, what is called *Ishana Shakti* in Sanskrit. It sets all forces in motion through currents that pervade everything.

Going over the mantra as a whole, section by section, **Ka E Ī La Hrīm** means desire (**Ka**), intention (**E**), motivation (**I**), fulfillment (**La**), **Hrīm**, the Shakti of light and realization. It sets our speech in motion as the Kundalini force to bring about the realization of the aspirations of our immortal soul.

Ha Sa Ka Ha La Hrīm indicates solar energy (**Ha**), lunar energy (**Sa**), desire (**Ka**), Prana (**Ha**), fulfillment (**La**), **Hrīm**. It sets our Prana in motion for the process of Self-realization.

Sa Ka La Hrīm reflects lunar energy as mind (**Sa**), desire (**Ka**), fulfillment (**La**), **Hrīm**, the Shakti of light and realization. It sets the mind in motion for the same process.

Sundari's mantras, including the Panchadashi, are not fiery or Kundalini mantras but Soma or watery mantras. They do not serve to directly stimulate or awaken the Kundalini force. But if the Kundalini force is awakened, they nourish, balance and guide it with the Soma on which it feeds. Along with the flow of Soma, these sounds stimulate the flow of inspiration in the mind, affording mantric and poetic powers to those who repeat them. They awaken the Kundalini force to merge into the crown chakra. In short, they contain the mantric key to higher consciousness within us.

The Panchadashi mantra is an important Soma mantra to help keep the Kundalini energy balanced as it rises. It increases Ojas, our primary vital energy reserve, and the mind's power to support and sustain the fiery electrical force of the Kundalini Shakti. This is the great importance of the Panchadashi mantra. Repeating it allows one to avoid the side-effects of unbalanced Kundalini energy.

Yet though this mantra is a benefic or soft mantra, it is still very powerful and should only be used with great caution by aspirants whose minds are clear and hearts are pure. If one wants to use the mantra, one should examine the entire worship of Tripura Sundari and the Sri Vidya, sincerely seeking grace and guidance both externally and internally from God and guru.

The Panchadashi mantra benefits from a conjoined usage of Kali mantras which serve to energize the Shakti in general, and

Bhairavi mantras which awaken the Kundalini. Whereas Sundari relates to the crown chakra, Kali relates to the heart chakra and Bhairavi to the root chakra. The three Goddesses cover the three primary chakras and through them the unfoldment of all the chakras.

Turning Kali into Sundari

Kali is the supreme Yoga Shakti in its unfoldment. Her energy arises with a relentless force and unstoppable movement, steadily driving us forward along our inner path. Yet over long practice, the power of Kali stabilizes, and becomes peaceful, gradually turning into the delight of Sundari. This transformation of Kali into Sundari is the essence of the inner Tantric Yoga, through which Shakti becomes bliss or Ananda.

We can facilitate this process with a few key mantras. First we begin with the prime threefold Kali mantra of **Krīm Hūm Hrīm**. To this we add the threefold Sundari mantra as **Aim Klīm Sauḥ**. To bridge the gap between the two we add the Devi mantra **Śrīm**. So the complete mantra is:

Om Krīm Hūm Hrīm Śrīm Aim Klīm Sauḥ

The Kali mantras, **Krīm Hūm Hrīm**, bring forth the Agni and Vayu or fire and air principles of energy. **Śrīm** softens the energy and makes it more nurturing. The Sundari mantras bring about the flow of Soma or bliss. This sevenfold mantra (eightfold if one counts the **OM**) combines the ascent of the Kali fire with the descent of the Sundari Soma. Once one has chanted the threefold Kali and Sundari mantras regularly for some time, one can take up this mantra and it will have power.

Tμe Goddess Bμairavi and tμe Kundalini Fire

Tantric Yoga is a powerful process of inner transformation, in which we raise our consciousness through all the levels of creation back to the Absolute that exists before and beyond every possible worlda, universe or state of mind. This inner transformation occurs through a special form of energy, which unfolds in its own dynamic and often unpredictable manner.

Tantric Yoga proceeds through the awakening of the *Kundalini Shakti* or 'serpent fire' in the root or Earth (Muladhara) Chakra at the base of the spine, where it lies dormant. The awakened Kundalini then ascends upwards through the chakras to the crown chakra or thousand petal lotus for the highest realization.

The question arises: How can we best facilitate the arousing of the Kundalini? How can we best relate to its extraordinary energy that can potentially short circuit our nervous system if we are not prepared to handle it?

The best way to approach the Kundalini is to recognize that it is the power and the presence of the Goddess within us. We must first honor and revere the Kundalini as a manifestation of the Divine Mother in order to unfold its energy in a truly harmonious manner. The best foundation for Kundalini Yoga is devotion to the Goddess,

161

which implies a connection with Shiva as well, though we might define or name these cosmic powers in different ways.

Kundalini is the highest manifestation of Shakti within our individual nature. It is the spiritual power of the soul, the portion of Divinity that we are in our deeper identity.[47] Kundalini supports the body and mind during our lifetime, sustaining even the autonomic reflexes in the physical body. Kundalini holds the potential for the development of higher consciousness within us. Honoring the Kundalini as a form of the Goddess ensures our proper relationship with her and the harmonious unfoldment of all our inner energies.

The Earth and Its Core Fire

Kundalini lies hidden in the Earth chakra, where in its state of sleep or latency it sustains our ordinary consciousness. To approach the Kundalini and the Goddess in general, we must first properly understand the root or Earth chakra, with which they are connected.

The root chakra is not simply the lowest of the chakras but the foundation of all the chakras. The root chakra is the seat of the Goddess within us; it represents Mother Nature and Mother Earth. As Earth or physical matter is the culmination of the universal creative process, the root or Earth chakra contains the potentials of all the worlds and their powers. It provides the ground, support and depth for our ascent to the Supreme.

Yoga practice is often defined according to the five elements and balancing them within us. As such, our Yoga practice should begin with making the Earth sacred within and around us. This means honoring the Earth in our natural environment, particularly in the soil, rocks and land forms and becoming aware of the presence of Shiva and Shakti within these natural formations. It means respecting our own physical body as a manifestation of the cosmic Earth element, our own rock or mountain designed to hold our soul's growths and developments in life.

With its emphasis on the secret power of the Earth, Tantric Yoga is inherently an ecological practice. It teaches us that our own natural environment is a manifestation of Shakti, the power of the Goddess, and carries her grace. To be able to reach up to the Heavens, we must first have our feet firmly planted on the ground. The summit of Heaven and the center of the Earth are one in an eternal mystical union! This is also the unity of the root chakra, our inner Earth, and the crown chakra, our mind's sky, and of Father Heaven and Mother Earth.

Hidden within the planet Earth is a secret power or Shakti of higher spiritual evolution. This Yoga Shakti is strongest in mountain regions like the Himalayas that allow the full power of the Earth element to be revealed. The same evolutionary power is hidden in the Earth of our own body, the root chakra, at the base of the mountain of the spine. Uncovering this mystical Earth within us is much like journeying into a secret cavern deep inside the ground, in which various gems or crystals can be found and holds a subterranean fire of enduring transformation.

However, these inner Earth powers are strong and primal and are not to be toyed with for mere personal gain or entertainment. They hold the primordial fires of life that like powerful currents of molten force can consume us. Existing even deeper than the roots of sexuality in Nature, these Earth currents hold the original will of the Divine to manifest in form, the soul's urge to embody itself in the field of physical matter. The secret space within the Earth holds the mystic foundry from which the soul can be transformed into the gold of pure awareness. We must approach these primal Earth energies with reverence in order to benefit from their energy, wisdom, vitality and grace.

The Goddess Bhairavi and the Root Chakra

The main Yogic Goddess who relates to the Kundalini fire is *Bhairavi*. She is a form of Shakti, specifically the marital or warrior aspect of Kali.[48] Bhairavi means 'fierce' or 'terrible'. She is the fierce form of fire that consumes the entire universe at the end of cosmic creation, dissolving it back into Pure Consciousness. Bhairavi dwells in a latent form in the Earth chakra and begins the yogic alchemical process from there.

We must learn to honor such fierce Earth Goddesses, like the volcanic fire beneath the Earth's crust that can erupt and shake the very foundations of our world. These Earth powers have their beauty and their fertility but they are awesome forces of nature that we cannot control at an individual or a societal level. The grace of the Goddess and the vision of Shiva are necessary for their proper development. Kundalini is a manifestation of a volcanic power within our own psyches. We should not attempt to arouse it unless we are well prepared to experience its force.

Bhairavi is also the main name for the Goddess in the Tantric traditions of Kashmir and Bengal. This is because of her identification with the fire energy which is the first power worshipped in the *Vedas*. Bhairavi is more than just the Earth fire; she represents all forms of fire culminating in the eternal and inextinguishable fire of Being itself (Brahmagni).

Vedic Yoga begins with the enkindling of Agni, the sacred fire on the Earth altar, which internally is the root chakra. As the *Upanishads* state, quoting the Vedic language, "First yogically controlling the mind, extending the inner intelligence, the Sun God, discerning the light of the fire, brought it forth from the Earth."[49]

Speech is the inner faculty that corresponds to fire in Vedic thought. In the yogic system, the supreme state of speech, *Paravak*, dwells in the root chakra. In this regard, the movement of the sound current is *downward* from the throat (manifest speech) to the heart (pranic speech) to the navel (illumined speech) to the root (transcendent speech).[50] Reaching the supreme level of speech, one also gains Self-realization and the awakening of all powers. By going to the inner essence of the root chakra as Divine Speech, one gains the capacity to open all the chakras.

This movement of the sound current down to the Earth complements and supports the movement of Prana up the spine to the crown chakra. It is the yogic descent that is the necessary balancing counterpart of the yogic ascent. Without this deeper descent, the real ascent is not possible. Without reaching the deepest, we cannot find the highest.

Bringing the fire out of the Earth is the first step of the inner Yoga. It requires bringing the soul (Jivatman), our inner fire, out of the wood or inert matter of our physical body. We must become conscious of our true Self at a soul level as a flame of awareness beyond the body and mind, working as a form of the Divine Fire on Earth to expand awareness, intelligence and delight.[51]

We must learn to contact the 'light of the Earth', the inner light of stone, the hidden Fire in the Earth and learn how to work with it. There is a fire in the Earth, which becomes stronger the deeper we go. A secret fire dwells at the core of the Earth not merely as a physical globe but as the hidden radiance behind our own body or physical mentality. This fire is not only primal but spiritual. It is the core fire of the soul that has created the earthly plane of existence and the human body for the purpose of Self-realization and union with the highest light. Matter is not simply dark but contains a Divine fire that can unfold matter into life and mind, in order to realize the pure consciousness of the Absolute beyond all time and space.

On a practical level, bringing the fire out of the Earth requires purifying the Earth of our body, which is the work of Ayurvedic medicine, in order to make the body a fit vehicle for receiving higher forces. Right diet and proper management of the digestive fire are the main means to do this. In addition, the practice of asana in Hatha Yoga is devised to stabilize the Earth element in the physical body so that it can serve as an altar on which the inner fire can be enkindled. The inner fire comes out through pranayama, which lifts the fire out of the Earth of the root chakra into the higher planes.

Awakening the Kundalini means awakening Bhairavi, the fierce and relentless aspect of Shakti that has entered into physical matter in order to mold and forge the life of the soul out of it. Bhairavi is an insatiable fire, driving spiritual growth, purification and transformation. She creates the inner desire and passion necessary to impel the soul upward into seeking something truly universal and fulfilling.

The Two Tripuras: Sundari and Bhairavi

Bhairavi is complementary to Sundari, as power is to beauty. They are the two aspects of the Goddess as harsh and soft, fire and water, Agni and Soma, and as the root and crown chakras. Shakti in the root chakra is Bhairavi, heating up the Prana and purifying us. Shakti in the crown chakra is Sundari, cooling the mind and bringing beauty and delight.

Bhairavi like Sundari is *Tripura,* which means 'having three forms,' relative to the three worlds of manifest existence as Earth, Atmosphere and Heaven and their three lights of Fire, Sun and Moon. These three forms also relate to the three aspects of our nature as Speech, Prana and Mind (Vak, Prana and Manas). Yet whereas Sundari represents the soft side of these three great powers, their beautiful light, Bhairavi carries their fierce side, their transforming heat.

Inner Tantric Yoga is a movement from Tripura Bhairavi to Tripura Sundari. It begins with the heat and pain of suffering, the practice of tapas and striving for the unknown. These are the fierce fires of Bhairavi, who causes us to seek the Supreme Shiva within us. It ends with the coolness and contentment of bliss, samadhi and Nirvana in the Absolute. This is the nectar of Sundari, who is ever in union with Shiva in their heavenly abode.

Bhairavi's Three Syllable Mantra

Bhairavi's three-syllable mantra develops out of the Sundari mantra of **Aim Klīṁ Sauḥ**, but with the additional pranic and fire sounds **H, S** and **R** added to them.

Hsraiṁ Hsklrīṁ Hsrauṁ

The pranic and fire sounds of **Ha, Sa** and **Ra** add tremendous energy and heat to the Sundari mantra, turning it from a soft soothing sound into a conflagration.

Because of its hot nature, Bhairavi's mantra should only be attempted with considerable care, caution, and the proper guidance. It should be used when seeking self-purification and not self-empowerment. It should be balanced with the mantras of Sundari for the complementary cooling force of Soma. One should always seek an integral development of Agni and Soma, the fierce and benefic forms, in order to guard against any excesses. If one has already activated benefic mantras like those of Sundari, one can gradually take up the mantra of Bhairavi.

Bhairavi's mantras activate the *Dakinis*, the special Shaktis of the chakras, particularly her mantra **Hsklrīm**. This consists of the sounds of *Hakini* (ha) for the third eye, *Sakini* (sa) for the throat chakra, *Kakini* (ka) for the heart chakra, *Lakini* (la) for the navel chakra and *Rakini* (ra) for the Sex Center. The Dakinis are the Yoginis that rule over the energies of the Chakras and should be propitiated in order to unfold their powers.

This mantra can be used in reverse order starting with the letter-**Ḍa**, which represents Dakini in the root chakra, as **Ḍrlkshaim**. Such mantras that consist mainly of consonants create a friction which can stimulate the Shaktis within us. To be able to pronounce this mantra, first add the vowel-a to each as **Da Ra La Ka Sa Haim**. Then try to eliminate the a-vowel so that only the consonants remain.

Combined with special pranayamas,[52] Bhairavi mantras can awaken the Kundalini fire dramatically and lift our consciousness upwards along with it. But for this to occur, we must first have our Earth or inner ground in the root chakra or we may just disturb our energies further.

Let us not forget the Earth or ground of our Yoga practice, which is to honor the Goddess powers of the Earth and make ourselves a fit vessel for them to work within us. For this we can worship the Earth as *Bhumi Devi*, the Earth Goddess, or as *Sita*, the consort of Lord Rama.

Another way to ground the Earth Chakra and the Kundalini force is to worship Ganesha there. One can use the mantra **OM Gam Gaṇeṣāya Namaḥ!** in the root chakra, or the single Ganesha bija mantra **Glaum**. Ganesha connects the Kundalini force with the deeper calmness of the higher mind.

Yet probably the most important consideration is always to worship the Goddess Durga before working with Bhairavi. Durga is the protective form of the Fire Goddess who removes all negativity, destroying all the anti-divine forces. Durga's mantra is:

Om Hrīm Śrīm Dum Durgāyai Namaḥ

One can also just use the initial three mantras, **Om Hrīm Śrīm Dūm**. While the force of Bhairavi, if awakened prematurely, can be harmful, Durga's energy is always benefic as long as we have devotion to her. She protects the Earth as the universal Mother. One can chant her mantra any time one wishes the grace and protection of the Goddess.

Drishti Yoga,
the Yoga of Perception

One of the most powerful and dynamic aspects of Tantric Yoga, but seldom extensively examined, is the 'Yoga of Perception', called *Drishti Yoga*. The use of the gaze, directed either outwardly and inwardly, can quickly and radically alter our consciousness and vitality. It can create a lightning like energy for increasing our Prana and developing a direct discriminating insight into the nature of Reality.

Along with mantra, pranayama and meditation, various techniques of holding or directing one's vision are important for awakening the higher energies of Yoga. As the eye is the guide of the body and the light of the mind, the Yoga of perception can be central for directing our practice. All serious students should include Drishti Yoga in their daily Yoga routine.

Yet the Yoga of perception is not an abstract or technical matter. Deities are part of the Yoga of perception just as they are part of other Yogas. Many deities—including several important Goddesses—reflect the secrets of the Yoga of perception, without which we cannot understand their functions or appearances. The Kundalini Shakti itself is a higher perceptual energy.

Drishti Yoga is closely connected to the practice of *dharana* or yogic concentration, which employs fixing the gaze on various inner or outer objects (antar drishti or bahir drishti). One common method of outwardly fixing the gaze is called *Trataka*, which consists of holding a steady gaze at the flame of a candle or ghee lamp. Various external objects can be similarly used for concentration, like looking at a tree or a flower and holding one's gaze upon them, allowing their energy to unfold within our minds.

We can also look at outer objects as manifestations of our own 'light of seeing' or *Drishti Shakti*. Outer objects can be brought into the inner gaze and we can experience them as formations of our own consciousness. The flame that we concentrate on externally can come alive and speak to us according to its role as the messenger of the Gods. We can discover the light of consciousness hidden in all that we see.

The internal fixing of the gaze consists of focusing on the chakras or other special places in the body like the tip of the nose or the point between the eyes. Fixing the gaze within not only concentrates the mind but draws our energy inward along with it, extending the action of pratyahara, or the yogic internalization of the prana and the senses.

An important dharana method is the 'Drishti of the five elements'. In this practice, one concentrates on an external form of the element and merges it inwardly into its ruling chakra, returning the outer aspects of the element into their inner origin in the subtle body.

- Focus your gaze on an outer form of the Earth element like a rock or a mountain and merge it inwardly into the root or Earth chakra at the base of the spine. Experience unity with all possible forms of the Earth element.
- Focus your gaze upon a river, lake or the ocean and merge the outer forms of the Water element into its inner origin in

the sex or Water chakra. Experience unity with all possible forms of the Water chakra.

- Focus your gaze on outer light forms like fire, a candle or the Sun and merge one's sense of light into the navel or Fire chakra. Experience unity with all possible forms of the Fire element.
- Focus your gaze upon clouds in the sky externally and merge the outer air into the inner Air or heart chakra. Experience unity with all possible forms of the Air element.
- Focus your gaze upon space externally and merge the outer space into the inner space of the throat or Ether chakra. Experience unity with all possible forms of the Ether element.

Yogic perceptual methods include internal visualizations, particularly visualization of the form of the deity or the form of its yantra. Each deity has its own meditation form (dhyana murti) with particular gestures, ornaments, weapons and attire that one meditates upon while invoking it.

Each deity has its yantra or geometrical form that reveals its internal energy pattern. Yantras are particularly important tools of the Yoga of perception. The Sri Yantra, for example, can be used as a perceptual devise for opening the crown chakra, the triangles of the yantra stimulating the petals of the chakra.

In addition, Drishti Yoga contains 'active perceptual exercises', like visualizing the very large in the very small and the very small in the very large. For example, one can imagine that a small rock is a large mountain or that a mountain is a small rock. This leads us to the eventual perception of the infinite in the finite and the finite in the infinite.

Another important perceptual method is to focus one's gaze on the space between objects and forget the objects themselves. This *Akasha Drishti* or 'gaze of space' opens up our higher awareness in a very powerful manner. Traditional Tantric texts like *Vijnana Bhai-*

rava contain many such perceptual methods. We have already discussed several of these in the second section of the book.

Importance of the Yoga of Perception

In the modern world, we are suffering from sensory disturbances that agitate our mind, emotions and prana. We suffer from an acute sensory overload through our media and computer-based culture. Yet behind this sensory excess is a greater sensory deprivation.

Our range of sensory impressions is severely limited by our technological culture. We no longer interact with or live in nature, which provides a much broader range of sensory stimuli that can help open deeper spiritual aspects of our minds and hearts, as well as link our prana with the cosmic life energy. We have lost our ability to appreciate the subtle hues of the Earth, the clouds and the sky, preferring the stronger but more uniform neon lights of our urban environment. The Yoga of perception creates a heightened inner sensitivity through which we can once more appreciate the beauty of all nature, as well as the spiritual energies hidden in our bodies and minds.

Such perceptual methods free our minds and senses from their conditioned responses, which are tied to how we direct our senses. Our perceptual patterns hold deep-seated emotional attachments, habits and addictions, which limit our ability to grow and develop inwardly in life. Yogic perceptual methods can help us undermine, circumvent and transcend these obstacles, bringing in new energy and a fresh vision. We can change our psychology radically, simply by changing how we look at the world and how we look at ourselves.

We must learn to use our perception creatively in order to consciously break out of our restrictive concepts of who we are and what the world is. Only then can we gain a window on the infinite and discover a new vision of Self and universe in which there is lasting peace and freedom. For an energetic Yoga practice to be complete, we must include the Yoga of perception, whether we perform special practices at certain times or generally hold our perception in an inner focus.

The Third Eye and the Power of Perception

The power of perception or *Drishti Shakti* is centered in the eyes, specifically in the third eye where the Lightning or Vidyut Shakti resides. It is the great Shakti force which sets in motion all other forms of Shakti. *This means that whatever we direct our gaze upon, we cast the lightning fire of perception upon it and energize it.*

If we focus our inner eye on the root chakra, we can aid in the awakening of the Kundalini fire residing there. If we focus our inner eye on the heart chakra, we can awaken the light of the inner Sun of pure awareness which abides there. If we focus our inner eye on the crown chakra, we can unfold the light of the inner Moon which relates to it and its currents of nectar.

This lightning perception of the third eye is also the weapon of the Gods. It is Shiva's glance that destroys *Kama Deva*, the God of desire. It is Indra's Vajra or lightning bolt that destroys the dragon of ignorance and releases the waters of immortal life to flow into the ocean of the heart.[53] This direct glance relates to the Goddess Chhinnamasta, who cuts off her own head by her sword of perception, revealing the infinite Void beyond the ego-mind.

To cultivate this direct power of perception, one focuses on an object directly, completely and with full attention. The light of perception then causes the object to open and reveal itself, becoming a doorway into the world beyond form, dissolving into the waves of consciousness.

Besides this fierce central gaze of Shakti is the 'side glance of Shakti' (Shakti kataksha), which is charming, attractive, and draws us into the inner light. The Goddess grants her side glance to her earnest devotees, bestowing on them her beauty, grace and abundance. We can cultivate this side glance by looking at things indirectly, drawing their attention to us, as it were, just as a beautiful woman need only cast a side glance on a man and need not look him directly in the eyes. The side glance opens the realms of subtle mystery, wisdom and energy, reflecting the allure of the unknown.

Drishti Shakti or the power of perception is a form of *Shakti-pat,* the giving of grace in Tantric initiations. The giving of Shakti through the eyes is probably the most powerful method of initiation. The direct lightning vision is harder to take and is only for more advanced devotees. The side glance is a more gentle way that stimulates the heart. Powerful Yogis all have strong Drishtis; the very power of their eyes draws us into their presence or darshana and is the basis of their charisma.

A special Tantric form of Drishti Yoga is to concentrate on the power of seeing as the reality. To do this, rather than directing our gaze towards a particularly object, one concentrates the power of seeing instead. One looks at the seeing instead of the objects seen. One meditates upon the light of perception as the reality, giving up one's fixation on the reality of the external world. One learns to contact, hold and direct the power of the eye like a ray of lightning. In this way, one's awareness merges into the perpetual lightning of inner perception.

Relative to Mantra Yoga, the I-sound relates to the Goddess and to perception as well, being the mantra of the eyes.[54] The mantra Īm stimulates perception in a direct manner, through either the outer physical eyes or the inner third eye. However, it is the destructive mantra Hūm, the sound of wrath, through which the destructive power of perception arises to remove negativities, as in the case of Shiva's gaze. The side-glance of the Goddess works through the mantra Klīm, which catches the mind and holds it with charm and grace.

Chinnamasta: The Eye Beyond the Mind

Kali is the great Goddess of Yoga, who assumes many different forms as the yogic process unfolds. Her fierce or powerful form is called 'Chandi', the red, wrathful or valorous aspect of the Goddess who destroys the negative forces, the Asuras or out of control life-energies that assail the practitioner. Bhairavi is a form of Chandi as the Kundalini Fire Goddess.

Kali's yet fiercer form is called 'Prachanda Chandi', the fierce or passionate form of Chandi. This is another name for *Chinnamasta*, which means 'a cut off head', probably the most unusual of the Goddesses, portrayed as drinking her own blood with her own head that she has just cut off!

Chinnamasta is also called *Vajra Vairochani*, 'who has the splendor of the diamond light', or *Vajra Yogini*, the 'diamond Yogini'. She is the great Yogini or Yoga Shakti of higher perception. The diamond or Vajra is the weapon of the great God Indra who represents the power of perception that can overcome all obstacles.

As the voluntarily cut off head, Chinnamasta represents the state beyond the mind, the entry into the void that occurs with the opening of the crown chakra. The opening of the crown chakra is often symbolized by a cut off head. It is the head, symbolizing the higher Self, which is released from the gross body. In the *Vedas*, the solar disc was regarded as a cut off head for this reason, the Divine light released from the world of form.

Chinnamasta is the power of Drishti Yoga, the Goddess as our guide along the Yoga of perception. She is Kali's power of lightning perception, the electrical force of the third eye. She is the eye behind the eye, the inner eye beyond the mind which is the perceptual power of the higher Self. This inner eye of the head is also the solar aspect of the crown chakra. The inner eye is both the seer of all and the consumer of all. It absorbs the entire universe into itself.

For Chinnamasta, one can use the mantra **Īm Krīm Hūm** for generating the lightning power of higher perception and discrimination. **Īm** is the power of seeing. **Krīm** is transformative electrical energy. **Hūm** is the expansion and explosion of pranic force and light. But again, use the mantra carefully and to purify and transform the mind and senses.

Shambhavi Mudra

Shambhavi mudra is a well known yogic practice that consists of focusing one's awareness within while looking outwardly through one's open eyes. Through the practice of Shambhavi mudra, the external world loses its solidity and is experienced in a vacuous form like clouds in space, without any fixed form or substance. The lightning fire of perception is directed within for the realization of Shiva or pure consciousness.

Practicing Shambhavi mudra is easy. It is best to do it while sitting, though one can do it while standing as well. Continue looking to the outside environment but steady your gaze and direct your attention within. Hold your gaze calmly and avoid blinking as much as you can. Concentrate inwardly on the pure light of Shiva, clear and transparent as the essential reality within and without. Yet while Shambhavi mudra is usually practiced with the eyes open, it can be done with the eyes half open or with the eyes closed. The important thing is the inner direction of the vision.

Shambhavi mudra is an important tool of concentration and meditation and probably the prime method of Drishti Yoga, from which many other methods are derived. Many Buddhist practitioners prefer to meditate in the manner as Shambhavi mudra with the eyes open, but the attention fixed within.

This same type of internalization practice can be used with all the senses. One can direct the attention within while the ears, skin, tongue or nose are engaged in their outward activities. A good way to do this is to focus on the inner aspect of the sense organ. For example, with the eyes, one can focus on the third eye or the right eye. With the ears one can focus on the right ear or the point at the top of the head. In this manner, one's attention goes into the power of the sense organ itself rather than the objects sensed by it.

Shambhavi mudra is a pratyahara practice, an interiorization of energy that is accomplished not by closing the senses, but by withdrawing the current of attention from the senses, even when they are active. One does not engage the senses or pursue their objects but holds one's awareness within. It is like holding one's attention in the depths of the sea even while sensing the waves at the surface.

Shambhavi mudra can be done with the Prana, directing it to the inner Self by holding the power of the breath. This 'inner fixing of the Prana' or *Prana-drishti* can be done in several ways. One can fix one's inner gaze on the heart as the seat of Prana. Another method is to fix one's gaze at the tip of the nose for the control of Prana, or at the point in space twelve fingers in distance from it. Or while performing pranayama, one can direct the Prana up and down the spine along with moving or rolling one's eyes, using the light of perception to stimulate the Kundalini force to ascend along with the breath.

Another form of Shambhavi mudra is to direct one's gaze inward to the heart, and through it merge the mind into the heart. You can hold your awareness in the spiritual heart, even while you are active outwardly through the body and senses. Keep your vision centered in the light of the heart whatever you do. In this way, you can transcend all the disturbances and fluctuations of the outer world. A related method is to unite the third eye with the eye of the heart. One can focus on the heart mantra **Hrīm** to aid in these processes.

The practice of Shambhavi mudra affords us deep peace in the midst of our hectic outer activities. This is particularly important today when few of us have any real time for ourselves or for doing any complicated yogic practices. Hold your center of gravity inside yourself and you will never fall into the pitfalls of life.

Looking Within to the Center of the Moon

One of the most important places of focus for the inner gaze is the soft palate at the back of the roof of the mouth. The soft palate is the juncture of all the five senses, where the mouth and the nasal passages meet along with their adjacent sinuses. The region of the soft palate is called 'the place of the Moon' in yogic thought. As the Moon relates to the mind in yogic symbolism, through concentrating at this point, the mind is easily is calmed.

In Vedic thought, the soft palate is the place where Indra or the higher power of perception is born, Indra-yoni. Fixing the gaze on the soft palate concentrates all the senses, opening the higher perceptive powers of the crown chakra through which one knows one's true Self.

The soft palate or place of the Moon is the womb of Shakti or *Shakti yoni* in the head, in which the powers of higher awareness are born. At this point one can experience all the rasas, the subtle essences, the tanmatras or subtle elements, the heavenly forms of sound, touch, sight, taste and smell, which provide the higher enjoyments of the heavenly worlds. From there the nectar or amrit, the Soma of the crown chakra flows downward. Fixing the gaze on the soft palate nourishes the Divine Child of higher perception within us. It allows higher secretions of inner contentment and deep relaxation to flow from the brain into the nervous system, relieving pain, anxiety and agitation.

This fixing of the gaze at the soft palate is an important means of energizing mantras. It works particularly well on Soma mantras, starting with the bija mantra **Śrīm** and extending to the Panchadashi mantra of the Goddess Sundari or her three syllable mantra **Aim Klīm Sauḥ**. Holding one's gaze at the place of the Moon while repeating such mantras affords the mantra more vitality and allows the Soma to flow through it. This is a great secret rarely revealed in yogic teachings.

The Gaze of Shiva and the Goddess Shambhavi

This looking within, whether the eyes are open or closed, is the 'gaze of Shiva' or *Shiva Drishti*. It reveals the presence of Shiva that pervades all things as the light of being. This gaze of Shiva is also the Goddess looking at Shiva. In this regard, Shambhavi is a form of the Goddess.

Shambhavi is the Goddess as the giver of the grace of perception. She is most closely connected to Sundari as her basic nature is beauty and beneficence. But she has a fierce side as well, which resembles Chinnamasta. The power of her gaze can remove any negativity directed towards us, through the lightning glance of her eyes. One can worship Ma Shambhavi to achieve the results of Shambhavi mudra and to gain the grace of Shiva.

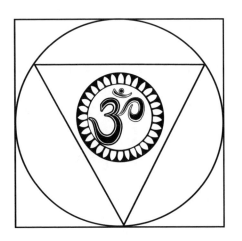

The Goddess Sati and the Power of Existence

Shakti is the prime fact of existence that is overflowing with intricate forces, intertwining currents and secret capacities known and unknown. Yet, perhaps strangely, the highest of all powers is the power of existence itself, not any outer force and its visible wonders. From the power of existence, like the root of a tree, all other forces of nature arise. It is the basis of life, love and light as the primary potentials of the soul.

Shakti is, first of all, the primal power of existence, not any outer or manifest force. The first Shakti is *Sat-Shakti*, the 'power or energy of Sat or Being'. The power of Being is the supreme energy, the beginning and the end of all powers, because it grants endurance to all things, holding them in the bosom of eternity. Without it nothing could last even for a second, and nothing could even be imagined.

From the power of existence arises time and all of its becoming, the movements of birth and death, creation and destruction. From its power of pervasiveness arises space and all the forms that manifest in space, all the elements and the worlds formed of them. From its all potential, a myriad different possibilities can be realized, understood and comprehended. Yet the power of existence is the highest of all possibilities, embracing all that we do.

181

The power of existence as Sat-Shakti gives rise to all the other Shaktis of consciousness, bliss, intelligence, mind, prana and body. It creates the electrical and propulsive forces of the universe by the effusion of its energy. It creates the magnetic and attractive forces of the universe by its ability to hold all things within itself.

The power of existence is the ground out of which duality, death, evil and suffering can arise. But it remains unchanging and untainted behind these negativities, which themselves can have no lasting reality. Evil cannot last even a day as the evil doer must return to the sleep of being in order even to function! The fullness of Being remains behind all other activities, however partial. When we recognize its power and follow its grace, all negativity can be transformed, not by any outer action but by Being itself.

The power of existence or Sat-Shakti is the supreme form of the Goddess, the supreme Shakti or *Parameshvari*. She is called *Gauri*, the white Goddess, with the color white symbolizing the purity of existence, who is Shiva's consort as pure as the snow of the white mountains from which she arises. The snow white mountain or Himalaya is itself a symbol of the power of pure existence which endures immobile through all outer changes. Shiva himself personifies pure existence, immutable, unmoving, full, stainless and independent. Shakti is the energy, grace and beneficent inherent within him.

The power of existence is also the 'power of peace', *Shanti-Shakti*. All higher powers arise from a deep inner peace, whereas the powers that stem from aggression, agitation or the effort to control are, if we look deeply, merely forms of weakness that bring about decay and fragmentation. The inner power of Being—which we can experience by holding to the power of the witness or the Seer within us—takes us beyond all outer disturbances, allowing our energy to be conserved and transformed. The power of peace is the highest power. It can neutralize all conflict and unite all positive forces. But to access it we must first of all have peace within our own minds and hearts, not merely peace as a social or political goal.

The Story of Sati

Sati as personifying the power of existence (Sat-Shakti) is said to be the first wife of the great God Shiva. According to the ancient story, Sati's father Daksha once wanted to perform a magnificent ritual and to it invited all the Gods, making lavish preparations for what he planned as his most glorious event. However, Daksha excluded Shiva and did not invite him, though Shiva was his own daughter's husband. This was owing to Shiva's unusual appearance and inability to follow the normal rules of behavior. To protest the dishonoring of her husband, Sati suddenly offered herself into the sacrificial fire at the beginning of this great ritual, giving up her own body.

This strange story possesses a deep inner meaning. Shiva as pure Being is transcendent. He is not a person, has no name and does not even possess a body. He is not part of the retinue of the other Gods, or even their ruler. He does not exist in the created world but has his abode only in the Absolute. No one can recognize him and he cannot be honored by anything external.

Daksha symbolizes the outgoing mind and its creative power, the ruling forces of the external world of duality. So he must by nature exclude Shiva whose reality is within. Daksha cannot even see Shiva because his gaze is inherently directed towards the outside. Sati symbolizes the power of the soul that in its inner purity is allied to Being or Shiva, but in its outer nature is part of the realm of Daksha or the outer world of Maya. The soul must sacrifice its involvement in the external realm and go beyond its conditioning in order to discover its real being. This is indicated by Sati's offering of her own body into the sacred fire. Sati is the power of Being within us that will not confine itself to the realm of becoming. In her essence, therefore, Sati herself has no body. As the power of existence, she must return to pure eternal existence beyond all manifestation, which is Shiva. Her reflection in time is but a shadow.

As the story continues, to avenge the death of his wife, Shiva and his retinue of spirits came and destroyed Daksha's sacrifice. This event similarly reflects a deeper meaning. Shiva's destruction of Daksha's sacrifice is Shiva's dissolution of the outer mind or intellect that Daksha represents. Shiva negates our outer vision of reality in order to draw us within to our true Self. He frees is from the rule of karma and rebirth, the cosmic order of the mind or Daksha, and takes us back to the Absolute. Once we come in contact with Shiva, all our preconceptions and cherished beliefs must go. He breaks down all our boundaries and attachments, particularly any kind of mere conformity to external influences, rules and customs.

Sati cannot really live in Daksha's world. She is the power of existence, the Shakti of Shiva that participates in but in essence transcends the manifest world. As the world develops outwardly, she must sacrifice herself and return to Shiva or the Absolute. Sati, like Shiva, can be represented as a corpse, meaning both are beyond time and action. Shiva and Sati rest as one, sleeping together, as it were, in eternal peace and delight. Theirs is the great night of eternity, *Maharatri*, where no thought or breath stirs. Theirs is the great day of eternity in which there is a perpetual dance of lightning, love and delight, without the need for any separate or manifest form.

We are all seeking to return to the power of existence, from which we have arisen and in which alone we can find our true home as a soul. In that supreme yet subtle and gentle force is our enduring Being beyond the vicissitudes of time and circumstances. We touch its realm of peace in deep sleep and it forms the foundation of all real samadhis or spiritual realizations. The soul ever wishes to return to its union with Shiva and Shakti as existence and power, as infinite Being permeated by unbounded energy, freedom and delight. This wish of the soul must be eventually fulfilled and all our different incarnations are but a seeking for it.

All grace comes from existence itself, from the very ground of Being that is our true nature in our deepest heart. We need not seek grace or even seek Being. We need only cease pursuing non-being, stop running after everything that does not reflect any real grace or carry any real essence.

The problem is that we do not yet really exist at a spiritual level. We do not dwell in our essential nature. We are caught in outer appearances and actions, in an endless becoming, seeking achievement or acquisition in the external world. This is the root of our ignorance and unhappiness which itself is not real. When we return to the power of Being, then all these problems disappear like stars before the rising Sun.

We fail to recognize the power of existence which is like space, silent and all-pervasiveness. We are hypnotized by the external powers of the world that are but shadows of the background force of being. Once we come into contact with the power of existence, all other powers get merged into it and we are no longer taken in by the external plays of the world or the illusions of the mind. We gain the force of our own being and become a presence to be reckoned with by all.

As the power of Being, the Goddess brings us back to Shiva who is Being itself. To be receptive to the power of Being as the grace of the Goddess is to really touch the heart of existence. Being is not an abstract idea or an unconscious force. It is the prime reality, Self-being, endowed with the supreme love and joy. It is the Mother of all.

To see Being as Shiva is to understand being in all of its fullness, which is not just the mere fact of existence, but being one with all and also being beyond all manifestation. That which is most transcendent is also that which is most primal and original.

The ground of existence is the highest goal of life and the highest state of awareness.

May we reclaim our Being and let go of all strife and striving in the realm of becoming. In that original state of rest, we naturally abide beyond birth and death, pleasure and pain. From that center, we can uphold all things and remain untouched and undisturbed by anything. Let us remember the power that we are, which gives strength and substance to all that has been, all that will be and all that is. We can do this with the great mantra of the supreme Brahman, **OM Tat Sat**!

PART FOUR

The Yoga of Shiva and Shakti

The Moon in the head, the Sun in the heart, Lightning in the eyes, Fire at the base of the spine, O Goddess, you dwell as the power of thinking in the head, as the power of seeing in the eyes, as the power of feeling in the heart, and as the power of light in the place of Fire.

GANAPATI MUNI, *INDRANI SAPTASHATI* 395–396

This section explains on the Yoga of Shiva and Shakti according to our internal energy centers. It is particularly important for practitioners relative to its yogic secrets, but the approaches indicated here can be helpful to anyone who wishes experience the inner light.

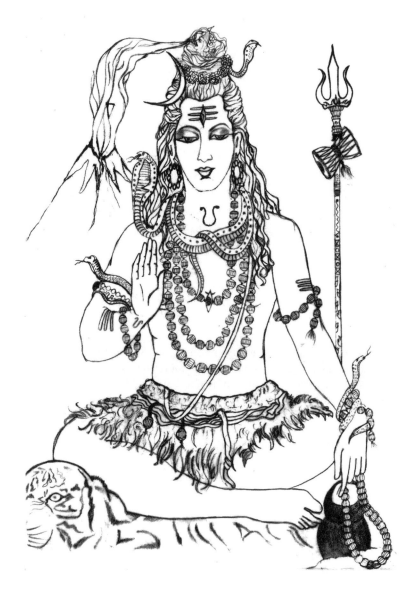

Shiva Maheshvara

Rudra and the Fire of Prana

Shiva is a deity of Prana, which is not only the life-force at a biological level but the universal principle of energy. This supreme
life-force is the basis of all manifestations of matter, energy and
mind. It is the first power of the higher Self, the Atman or Purusha.
If we wish to return to the Self, Prana shows us the way back.

The inner practice of Yoga revolves around working with Prana on all levels of body, mind and spirit. Ayurvedic medicine is
based upon employing the power of Prana as the primary healing
force behind all of its therapies. Vedic astrology reflects the connection between Prana and light and the dispensation of karma
through the cycles of life. Prana has control over all activities in
the universe and all the movements of the mind, emotions and
senses. Prana is the main Yoga Shakti or power of Yoga. Even the
Kundalini Shakti is the awakened Prana of the soul. The Devi as
Shakti is the essence of Prana and grants unbounded vitality to her
devotees.

Prana has its own form of Agni or fire called the *Pranagni*, the
'fire of Prana', which works behind the breath, our internal organs, our sense and motor organs. The fire of Prana is responsible
for sustaining life at an autonomic level, stimulating the nervous

system and maintaining the digestive fire, though which homeostasis occurs.

This fire of Prana relates to the deity *Rudra*, the fierce form of Shiva. Rudra is the source of all healing powers and grants rejuvenation and revitalization to both body and mind. We contact the transformative energy of Rudra whenever we undergo a catharsis in life, whether it is an emotional change of heart that brings about a major shift in our personality, or a healing crisis that causes the body to detoxify itself. Rudra is always present within us to bring greater intensity into our lives, whether we like it or not, as that intensity is what causes us to grow and evolve.

This fire of Prana is ultimately the energy of all life and existence. At a cosmic level, Rudra is the universal Prana personified, the *Prana Purusha*, the 'Self' or 'soul of Prana'. This deeper Prana sustains us during the state of deep sleep when the mind and the senses are at rest. The same Prana takes the soul after death to higher worlds and on to its next birth.

Prana has its own intelligence that goes far beyond our personal intellect, of which the natural intelligence of the body is but an outer aspect. This natural intelligence of Prana sustains both instinct and intuition within us, maintaining our organic equilibrium at a subconscious level and developing our spiritual potential at a superconscious level.

The Pranic fire has a lightning or electrical nature, acting suddenly, fiercely, unpredictably and relentlessly. It can reawaken life and feeling within those who are dull and can even revive the dead or dying. Yet, as a destructive force, Shiva's fire becomes the lightning that is the 'weapon of the Gods,' which destroys all undivine and disharmonious forces. Many ancient Vedic mantras reverberate with a supplication to Rudra to turn his arrow away from us and protect us from his wrath.[55]

Rudra's arrow is the power of the universal Prana that can raise our life-energy when we unite with its ascending current, or cut off our life-energy when we go against its indomitable will. Death is not the denial of life but the life-force leaving the body for a more suitable form of manifestation. Rudra facilitates the healing and transformation that is both life and death.

The Pranic Fire and Mantra

The main ways to work with the pranic fire are through pranayama, mantra and meditation. Here we will focus on the mantra as the inner key. Mantra holds a pranic power of speech from its connection to the outgoing breath. The *Vedas* tell us that *Prana is unmanifest speech, while speech is manifest Prana*. We speak through the outgoing breath and can inhale only when we are not speaking. All mantras and sounds of the Sanskrit alphabet arise through Shiva's drum. They are forms of Shiva, beginning with the **OM**, which is his power of expression.

More specifically, there are certain 'pranic sounds' in the alphabet which serve to connect speech and breath. 'S-sounds' and 'h-sounds', or what are called 'sibilants' in linguistic terms, relate to Prana and its fire. They are called *ushmas* in Sanskrit or 'what produces heat'. They reflect the natural sound of the breath and intensify it further, adding the power of the mind to it. We find these pranic sounds in mantras like **So'ham** or **Hamsaḥ**, the sounds of the breath through inhalation and exhalation.[56]

An excellent mantra for Pranagni, the Pranic fire or Rudra to prepare the Soma, the nectar of the higher mind and brain, is:

OM Hrīm Krīm Hūm Hamsaḥ So'ham Svāhā!

The mantra **OM** refers to the unmanifest Prana that is one with the Absolute. **Hrīm** is the inner or seed Prana of the heart and the basis of creation. **Krīm** brings about the activation of the electrical force of Prana into manifestation. **Hūm** reflects the expansive aspect of Prana as light and fire. **Hamsaḥ** and **So'ham** represent the fiery and watery aspects of Prana or the solar and lunar, projective and reflective aspects of light. **Svāhā** is the mantra of consecration to the cosmic fire.

Use this mantra before you start your practices of pranayama or meditation in order to energize the Prana within you, repeating it for a few minutes with a soft voice or silently in your mind. You can repeat the first four bijas on inhalation, **Om Hrīm Krīm Hūm**, and the remaining bijas on exhalation, **Hamsah So'ham Svāhā!**

The deity Rudra is the *Paramahamsa,* the most supreme (parama) liberated soul or pranic being (hamsa), the one whose life-energy and soul has moved beyond all limitations of body and mind. His pranic power invigorates the body and opens the deeper mind and heart. It grants us the energy of *tapas* and *tejas*, the inner heat of spiritual fervor and aspiration; the courage, fearlessness and boldness to break through our human attachments and merge into the Cosmic Being. The Paramahamsa is one who breathes with the unbreathing breath of the Infinite Brahman and its Supreme Light (Paramjyoti).

We must arouse that fearless and focused Rudra energy within ourselves if we wish to reach a state of deep transformation. For this to occur, we must be willing to be bold and adventurous—to dare to risk our lives as it were—to challenge the boundaries of ordinary human consciousness and move into the great Unknown. Only those who unwaveringly can take up the stern challenge of Rudra can reach the supreme goal of Life, in which birth and death dissolve into a power beyond description, dwarfing the creation of all the universes and engulfing the energies of all time and space. While our initial contact with Rudra may be harsh, in the long run he will become our best friend and most certain guide, who never bows down to the opinions of the human mind or to the likes and dislikes of anyone.

Maha Mrityunjaya Mantra

The most famous and oldest of the chants to Shiva is the *Maha Mrityunjaya Mantra* from the *Rig Veda (VII.61.12)*, which is attributed to the Rishi Vasishta, the most famous of all the Vedic seers. It means the great (maha) means of conquering (jaya) death (mrityu). It is also called the *Trayambakam Mantra* after its first word, Trayambakam, the three-eyed One, referring to Rudra-Shiva.

The Maha Mrityunjaya Mantra is the most important Vedic mantra for healing body and mind and for dealing with all negativity and suffering possible in life, whether from other people, wild animals, the forces of nature or spiritual forces. It is a great mantric hymn to Rudra-Shiva as the personification of the *Yajna*, the Vedic sacrifice, which outwardly is the karmic movement of the universe, and inwardly is the yogic movement of the transformation of the mind and heart from darkness to light. Reciting this chant helps us remove negative karmas in life—particularly those owing to the planetary influences of the malefic planet Saturn—and also promotes the awakening of the Kundalini or higher Pranic fire.

**Tryambakam yajāmahe sugandhim puṣṭivardhanam
Urvārukam iva bandhanāt mṛtyor mukṣīya māmṛtāt**

*We worship the Three Eyed One whose fragrance is beautiful
and who is the increaser of nourishment. Like a cucumber from
its stalk, release us from death but not from immortality!*

This powerful mantra reflects our organic connection with the Supreme. Shiva is present in the beautiful fragrances of our life-experience, the soul essences that we imbibe when we feel things deeply in our hearts. He increases our ability to draw nourishment from both life's blessings and tragedies. This inner feeding of the soul gradually ripens it over time. Then it can naturally leave the field of mortality and enter the realm of immortality, just as a ripe cucumber can fall off the vine without any strain or effort. God-realization is present within us, like a seed, as the higher organic potential of the soul. We need only tend to it with the light of meditation, the water of devotion, and the soil of service and it will grow into divinity in its own time and manner.

While this mantra is commonly used, there are three important bija mantras that make it much more powerful, which are not as well known. They make the mantra much more effective and can also be used by themselves for the same healing and saving purposes.

OM Haum Jūm Saḥ!

- **Haum** is perhaps the most important bija mantra for Shiva. It is **Aum** plus the pranic sound **H**, or **OM** in its full pranic energization. As such, the mantra grants strength, awareness and vitality that is unlimited.
- **Jūm** (pronounced joom) is the main bija mantra for quick healing and saving action. The root 'ja' indicates movement, speed, velocity, vitality and generative powers. The vowel-**u** adds energy, strength and protective power to it. We can compare the bija **Jūm** with **Hūm**. **Hūm** increases the power of Prana in a fiery and expansive manner that can be creative or destructive. **Jūm** increases the speed, agility and instantaneous healing ability that arise from Prana.
- **Saḥ** refers to the Being, Self, Atman or Purusha, our higher nature. The formula, **OM Haum Jūm Saḥ**, works to create pranic energy and to direct it towards healing and protecting the Being or Self. **Saḥ** also serves to hold the energy generated by **Haum Jūm**.

One can repeat the mantra forward and backwards for additional power, either by itself or before and after the Mrityunjaya mantra.

OM Haum Jūm Saḥ, Saḥ Jūm Haum OM

Repeat this mantra, **OM Haum Jūm Saḥ**, for a few minutes whenever you need additional energy, vitality or healing power, remembering Lord Shiva as the supreme Prana and power of rejuvenation. Let your breath naturally deepen and vitalize the heart as you use the mantra.

How to Manifest the Deity: Prana Mantras

The force of Prana relates not only to s and h-sounds (sibilants), but also to what are called 'semi-vowels', the letters **Y, R, L, V** or the Sanskrit syllables **Ya, Ra, La,** and **Va.** Intermediating between vowels and consonants in their energetic quality, semi-vowels reflect the Prana or energy that mediates between the formless realm and the realm of form, the Divine and the world.[57]

These Prana mantras are employed in an important process called *Prana-Pratishta,* 'establishing the life or the spirit', an extraordinary ritual performed in Hindu temples in order to bring the actual spirit of the deity into the forms used for worship. According to Hindu thought, without first installing the spirit of the Deity into the image, the image has no power and is only a material form, but when the spirit of the Deity brought into it, the image can serve as a conduit for the Deity and all of its majesty and wisdom.

The most common Prana-Pratishta mantra is as follows:

Om Ām Hrīm Krom Yam Ram Lam Vam Śam Ṣam Sam Ham
Kṣam Hamsaḥ So'ham

To these bija mantras, a mantra for the deity, either Shiva or the Goddess is added:

Śivasya Jīva iha sthitaḥ, meaning "May Shiva's living soul dwell here."

Devyāḥ Jīva iha sthitaḥ, meaning "May the living soul of the Goddess dwell here."

The mantras **OM Ām Hrīm Krom** serve to call the Divine power down into the form. **OM** opens the energy. **Ām** expands the energy. **Hrīm** draws the energy into the heart. **Krom** adds an intensity of feeling and emotion. The four semivowels (**ya, ra, la, va**) and five sibilants (**śa, ṣa, sa, ha, kṣa**) bring the image to life, awakening its Prana and senses.[58] **Hamsaḥ So'ham** brings in the Spirit, Self or soul of the deity.

The same process of drawing down the Deity can be used on ourselves, to invoke the living spirit of the Deity into our minds and hearts, to bring Shiva and Devi to life within us! We should install the Divine Prana not only in outer forms of worship but in our own bodies as the inner form of worship. Yet this is not something we can do quickly or casually. It is not our ego-self that is to be exalted. First the ego-self must be dissolved. The open egoless mind and heart is the receptacle necessary to invoke the deity within us.

For this purpose, first empty your mind of all desire, fear, striving and seeking. Let go of your personal self and its psychological conditions. Ready your inner being to enter into the Eternal. Then meditate upon the Divine in the form or aspect of your choice, visualizing the deity as dwelling in the eight–petal lotus of the spiritual heart that reflects all the directions of space.

Then use these Prana Pratishta mantras to draw the spirit of the Deity into you as your true immortal Self. Repeat the mantras seven times to bring the deity into all of your chakras. Then rest in the presence of the Deity, letting the world dissolve into the Infinite sea of Awareness. When your mind resurfaces, strive to hold the memory of the Deity within you as your true nature.

The Four Inner Lights
and Energy Centers

Spiritual practice is all about light; bringing in the light and, most importantly, moving from darkness to light. Yoga is primarily an inner science of light, with its various aspects, from asana to meditation, simply different methods of cultivating the higher light within us.

Shiva as the Supreme Deity is defined as pure light, *Prakasha*. He indicates the original clear light of consciousness behind all light forms in the universe. Shakti is the energy that arises from this original pure light as the lightning of perception, life and expression.

This 'inner light' is not just a metaphor but can be experienced quite vividly by the meditative mind. The inner light is the supreme light beyond all outer forms of light, transcending all dualities of light and darkness in the external world. It exists prior to and beyond the five elements of Earth, Water, Fire, Air and Ether, including beyond light or fire as an element. This inner light of Being endows brilliance to the light of the Sun, beauty to the light of the Moon, and color to the light of Fire. At an inner level, it grants the light of understanding to the mind and energy to Prana.

197

This inner light is not just an idea or emotion but the ultimate power behind our faculties of speech, prana, sight and mind. It has different forms, functions and locations within us that we can experience as the basis of higher Yoga practices. In this regard, there are four main centers of light in the body and the chakras: 1) The region of Fire or Agni, 2) The region of the Sun or Wind, Surya or Vayu, 3) The region of the Moon or Soma, 4) The region of Lightning or Vidyut.

These regions are so named because they carry a type of energy similar to the corresponding light forms in the external world of nature. But we should not literally identify them with their outer counterparts. They are far more subtle than these external forms of light, holding a life and intelligence that we can communicate with inside ourselves. The Fire within us, for example, is a life fire and a soul fire, not a simple material fire as in the external world.

- **The region of fire or Agni** relates to the three lower chakras of the root, sex and navel centers and to the digestive fire (*Jatharagni* in Ayurvedic medicine). Its main center is the root chakra where it dwells as the Kundalini Shakti.

  Its ruling deity is Bhairavi among the great Goddesses. It relates to the higher energy of Pitta or the biological fire humor in Ayurvedic medicine and its subtle essence as *Tejas* or inner radiance.
- **The region of the Sun (the gaseous fire) or Wind** relates to the three middle chakras of Navel, Heart and Throat, but particularly the Heart, which is the seat of the air element, and to the fire of the breath, the 'Pranic fire' or *Pranagni*. It also relates to the spiritual heart (hridaya) that is beyond all the chakras. Vayu or Wind is the expansive aspect of this energy, which is also the wind of space, not just the atmospheric wind, while the Sun is its inner center as the supreme Light of lights.

Its ruling deity is Kali among the great Goddesses, particularly in its Vayu aspect. It relates to the higher energy of Vata or the biological air humor in Ayurveda and its subtle essence as Prana or inner vitality.

- **The region of the Moon** relates to the three higher chakras of the Throat, third eye and head or crown chakra, but specifically to the crown chakra, which is the region of the mind and relates to the Moon in Vedic thought.

  Its ruling deity is Sundari among the great Goddesses. It relates to the higher energy of Kapha or the biological water humor in Ayurveda and its subtle essence as Ojas or the inner power of patient endurance.

- **The region of Lightning** is that of the third eye and the fire of the mind specifically, and the fires of perception and discrimination. Its ruling deity is Chinnamasta among the great Goddesses, the more fierce form of Kali. It relates to perceptive power of Pitta or the biological fire in Ayurveda and our Buddhi or higher discriminating intelligence.

The Yogic Alchemy of Light

Tantric Yoga—like the Vedic Yoga out of which it developed—revolves around the 'union of Agni and Soma', the fire and the moon, or the Kundalini and Soma powers. In this process, the Kundalini fire ascends up the spine from the root chakra causing the Soma in the crown chakra to melt and drip down throughout the body and opening the other chakras along the way.

In Tantric symbolism, Agni represents the feminine principle or Shakti, which relates to the female reproductive fluid and menstrual blood that is red in color and possesses a heating and fiery nature. Soma indicates the masculine principle or Shiva, which relates to the semen that is white in color and possesses a cooling and lunar nature.

However, the polarity of the reproductive system is opposite to the polarity of the body as a whole. In the body overall, the female principle is Soma or water and the male is Agni or fire. That is why women have more body fat and water and a cooler nature, while men have a hotter and more aggressive temperament. But in sexuality and inner Yoga practices the polarity gets reversed.

The union of Agni and Soma results in the development of Surya, the solar force, and Vayu as the great Prana, its wind of light or expression. The ascending fire and descending nectar allow the light and energy of the heart to expand.

The lightning of the third eye serves as the spark, the lighter or the trigger for the other three lights to manifest, just as lightning causes fire to arise on the Earth when it strikes dry vegetation the ground. The lightning force underlies the other three forces as the prime Shakti. It is the inner lightning that arises from space and clarity in the mind.

Each of these four energy centers relates to a particular function of our nature and has special Yoga practices to go along with it:

- Agni or fire relates to the faculty of speech, both as a motor organ and as the capacity of the mind to express itself, and to the practice of mantra or *Mantra Yoga*.
- Surya or the Sun relates to Prana and the practice of pranayama or *Prana Yoga* at an outer level, and to the inner Self or Atman and *Jnana Yoga*, the Yoga of Knowledge and Self-inquiry, at an inner level.
- Soma or the Moon relates to the mind and to the practice of meditation, particularly of a reflective or contemplative nature or *Dhyana Yoga*, which has both devotional and knowledge-oriented approaches.
- Vidyut or Lightning relates the eye and to our perceptual capacities in general, and to yogic perceptual methods of fixing the gaze inwardly and outwardly or *Drishti Yoga*.

Yet mantras can be used for all four energy centers.

- Agni or the Fire of the root chakra is energized by fiery mantras, notably **Hūm**, but also **Hsraiṁ Hsklrīṁ Hsrauṁ**, Bhairavi Mantras and Durga mantras like **Hrīm Śrīm Hūm**.
- Surya or the Sun of the Heart is energized by solar mantras, notably **Hrīm**,[59] while the Wind force is energized by pranic mantras like those of Kali, **Krīm Hūm Hrīm**.
- Vidyut or the lightning of the third eye is energized by lightning mantras, notable **Krīm**, but also **Īm** and Chinnamasta mantras like **Hūm**.
- Soma or the Moon of the crown chakra is energized by lunar mantras, notably **Śrīm**, and Sundari Mantras like the Panchadasi Mantra and **Aim Klīṁ Sauḥ**.

The Vedic approach emphasizes these four centers as aspects of the Purusha, the Cosmic Being or Shiva principle, the light of consciousness. This is the basis of the ancient Vedic Yoga. The Tantric approach emphasizes these four centers as aspects of the Devi, the Cosmic Energy or Shakti principle, the energy of consciousness. This is the basis of the inner Tantric Yoga. But the understanding of the four centers and their processes continues from the Vedic to the Tantric, which employ similar mantras, deities and practices in order to work with them.

Besides needing to raise the Kundalini fire to the crown chakra, we also need to strengthen each of these four centers in their own right.

- We need to increase and expand the coolness, reflective light, calm and contentment of the Moon of the mind and the crown chakra in order to allow for our awareness to function at a deeper level.
- We need to increase the energy of Lightning as the percep-

tual power of the third eye in order to awaken our higher powers of seeing and discrimination.

- We need to expand the light and warmth of the Sun in the heart in order to open up our deeper sense of Self, our feelings of unity, and a greater power of Prana.
- We need to increase the power of Fire in the navel in order to develop a greater energy of speech that can project all the powers of creation starting from the Earth itself.

Besides representing four different centers, these four powers can be used to work on any of the seven chakras.

- The light of the Moon serves to cool, calm and nourish each chakra we direct it towards, through the light of the reflective mind and its power of bliss, peace and contentment. Contemplative forms of meditation, like meditation on universal peace or eternal love, can be used on all the chakras for this calming purpose.
- The light of Lightning serves to awaken each chakra through its powerful electrical and pranic force of Pure Consciousness. A one-pointed gaze or lightning power of visual perception can be focused on any chakra for this stimulating purpose.
- The light of the Sun serves to fully open each chakra through the power of the higher Prana and the awareness of the higher Self. We can direct the solar force of Prana through the breath to any of the chakras in order to expand its energy, or we can use the solar force to bring the awareness of the universal Self to each chakra and the factors it rules over.
- The light of Fire serves to energize each chakra through the power of mantra at the level of primal sound. Fire mantras like **Hūm** can be used on all the chakras for this purpose, to increase their respective inner fires.

The prime mantras for these four lights can also be used in the different chakras and energy centers.

- **Krīm** can be used to energize all the chakras with the electrical force of lightning perception.
- **Hūm** can be used to empower all the chakras with expansive heat and strength.
- **Hrīm** can be used to fill all the chakras with radiance and space.
- **Śrīm** can be used to nurture all the chakras and provide them bliss and delight.

Usually the movement of Tantric Yoga is explained relative to the ascent of the Kundalini fire, but we must recognize that all four centers and their light powers play important roles. In this regard, we must recognize that the Kundalini fire, when properly developed, is not a destructive fire. We can better understand it relative to the force of electricity. Electricity in itself is very hot and, if we do not ground it properly, it can shock and burn us to death if we touch its current directly. But in the proper channels, electricity is a force that can run any number of appliances, even those that are cooling like a refrigerator or an air conditioner. *When we keep the Kundalini flowing in the proper channels it can unfold the powers of all the chakras and all four light centers.*

As the Kundalini fire rises, it does not simply increase heat, it energizes all the light centers that it awakens. It allows for the full expansion of the light of the Moon in the head. It allows for the full expansion of the light of the Sun in the heart. It allows for the full power of the Lightning of perception in the third eye. And it sustains its own primal Fire of life and existence in the root chakra below.

Developing these four powers of light is central to the inner yogic alchemy. It requires deep dedication, concentration and a steady application of effort and attention. As the higher chakra forces unfold, they connect us with the greater wonders of the conscious universe that even modern science has yet to imagine, and a beauty and bliss that is beyond all formulation or expression.

Become aware of these four lights, four energies and four centers within yourself and begin to work with their powers as the light and energy of your own being. To facilitate this process, recognize that light is the Purusha or Cosmic Self and energy is the Goddess. Be a light and power unto yourself not as a separate principle but as the source and support of all that is. Become the inner light of the Supreme God within you and the inner energy of the Supreme Goddess.

The Supreme Light of Shiva

At the highest level, one can merge into the clear light of Shiva behind all four great light powers. Great Jnanis, masters of the Yoga of Knowledge, can go directly to the light of Shiva, and integrate all light, energy and knowledge into it. The clear light of the Absolute holds the bliss of the Moon, the insight of Lighting, the radiance of the Sun and the heat of Fire as one single reality.

Chant '**OM Namaḥ Śivāya!**'[60] and enter into the light of Shiva that is the crystal light of Being-Consciousness-Bliss! Become one with the presence of the light of Shiva that is the very essence of all that is, has been or is yet to be!

Soma and the Yoga of the Crown Chakra

The highest Soma vessel is the crown chakra or thousand petal lotus, from which the nectar of immortality flows. This vessel of the head is ultimately drunk by the Self, God or Atman in the heart, who in the process consumes all our desires and transmutes them into bliss.

Yet this drinking of the Soma is the result of a long practice that has several stages and does not happen quickly. The nectar of the crown chakra requires the insight of the third eye to open it up, the development of Prana expand it, and the Kundalini fire to ripen it.

The prepared nectar or open crown chakra is often symbolized as the head that has been cut off, representing the 'no-mind' state. Opening the crown chakra requires going beyond the ordinary head or ordinary mind to the spiritual head which is infinite space. Deities who have had their heads cut off are common in Tantric and Vedic traditions reflecting this great truth of the no-mind condition. The ancients often looked upon the round spheres of the Sun and the Moon as heads that were cut off. The cut off head symbolizes the soul liberated from the Samsara of embodied existence into pure awareness!

205

The main Tantric deity showing this headless state is the Goddess Chinnamasta. In her case, she drinks the blood gushing from her severed neck with the cut off head that she holds in one hand, carrying the sword that she used to cut her head off with in the other hand! Her frightful image is not the product of some dark superstition but indicates the mystic death and transformation that accompanies the opening of the crown chakra.

Ultimately, we must offer our heads, meaning our conditioned minds, in sacrifice to the inner divinity. Man is the Soma for the Gods as the *Vedas* say. One must offer one's head or crown chakra, as a full vessel to the Gods for their enjoyment, who will drink it, turning us into Gods in the process. Though we may find this metaphor to be a bit graphic, for those who have gone beyond life and death, it quite clearly represents the intensity of their experience.

Chinnamasta with her severed head shows the action of the third eye to open the crown chakra. She indicates the discriminating insight that can extract the Soma from all our life experiences, good and bad, happy and sad. On the other hand, Sundari, the great Goddess of beauty and delight, shows the drinking of the Soma from the open crown chakra, which results in the bliss and beauty of Divine perception.

This means that Sundari or Divine bliss is not possible without Chinnamasta, the mystic death and self-sacrifice. Chinnamasta indicates the open crown chakra or head, drinking the blood of our life experiences, which she converts into Soma. The nectar of immortality must be prepared by drinking one's own blood and consuming all our mortal desires. We must learn to extract the Soma of bliss from the blood of desire.

The Yoga of the Crown Chakra

The yogic process for developing the nectar of the crown chakra is very interesting. *First, the elixir in the head must be prepared.* In the ordinary human being, the crown chakra is contaminated with forces of ignorance, darkness and confusion. To prepare it as an elixir, our vital energies must be purified and drawn up to the head, through processes of meditation, mantra and pranayama. The bliss from our lower emotional impulses must be extracted and raised to the head, not simply to the brain but to the mind of the soul, where it can be dissolved into Divine contemplation.

To prepare the inner nectar, we must make the mind an effective vessel to hold it, so that the nectar can consolidate. There is a very simple approach to this: *For the inner Yoga or even for ordinary psychological well-being, we first need to cool down the mind.*

Our ordinary state of mind is overheated, over stimulated and over agitated. We react quickly to things, 'losing our cool' and along with it the mind loses its basic calm nature and falls into disturbance and sorrow. We lose the inner nectar or Soma of contentment inherent in the mind and get caught in the pleasures of the outer world for our sense of well-being, which must eventually prove illusive.

The cool mind alone is able to hold the nectar of bliss and rejuvenation within us. Coolness of mind is the basis of peace and detachment. An inwardly cool mind does not attach itself easily to external phenomenon as it is already content and at ease within itself. Nothing can disturb it or influence it from the outside.

Most importantly in Yoga, *a cool mind is necessary to handle the heat and energy of the Kundalini Shakti. Before we seek to raise the Kundalini fire we must first cool down the mind.* This requires giving up the anger, aggression, and opinionated nature of the egoistic mind and the critical intellect that thinks it already knows everything. It requires the mind to let go of its idea of the reality of the outer world and embraces the inner reality of Consciousness.

To keep our minds cool, we must turn our mental and pranic energy within, reflecting the Divine Self inside us, rather than pursuing the enjoyments of the external world. We should let our attention flow within and cease worrying about the external world and its endless fluctuations.

To cool down the mind, we must also slow it down. To do this we must reduce our rate of sensory activity, withdrawing from the rapid media stimulation that our modern culture promotes to a deep contemplation of the world of Nature and the unbounded voidness of space. We must remember to keep the Fire in the belly and the Moon or coolness in the head and mind.

Soma Pranayama

The upward movement of the Kundalini is associated with the breath and certain special breathing practices or pranayamas. In such 'Kundalini fire pranayamas', one visualizes the inner Fire or Kundalini ascending to the crown chakra during inhalation, its rising heat causing the Soma in the crown chakra to melt. Then the Soma descends upon exhalation, bringing its cooling energy down to the heart and the entire body. This approach serves to heat up the energy in the head and expand one's awareness ultimately into the Void.

Yet there is a complementary 'lunar pranayama' that involves the ascent of the Moon and the descent of the Sun. There is an ascending lunar pranic current that we can energize through the process of inhalation, which cools and calms the mind, brain and senses. This current is called *Apana Chandra* in Tantric thought, or the 'apana or watery Moon breath', as in the works of the great Kashmiri Tantric Abhinavagupta.[61]

One draws the mind up the spine during inhalation as a cooling energy, merging it into the crown chakra and using it to increase the Soma. To create this cooling energy one breathes in through the mouth, with the tongue held at the roof of the mouth in order to draw the energy further upwards.

After inhalation is over, one brings the light down from the head on exhalation, particularly the lightning from the third eye, to stimulate the Kundalini Fire in the root chakra. This exhalation is the *Prana Surya* or 'solar Prana' in Tantric thought. For this one places the tongue back to its usual position at the bottom of the mouth, in order to protect the energy above.

To facilitate this pranayama, one can use the natural mantras of the breath, mentally repeating the sound **So** on inhalation, which in Yoga has a cooling or lunar nature, and the sound **Ham** on exhalation, which in Yoga has a heating or solar nature. Alternatively, one can use the lunar Shakti mantra **Śrīm** on inhalation and the solar Shakti mantra **Hrīm** on exhalation. In any case, one should let the breath naturally deepen and the mind naturally expand in a reflective and contemplative mode.

To facilitate this pranayama yet further, one can visualize one's own awareness entering into the Moon of the mind, appearing like a small white drop (called bindu in Sanskrit) and through this drop bring one's awareness up the spine like the Moon rising in the sky. On exhalation, one can visualize the energy of the lightning fire descending from the third eye but along with the expanse of Soma or rain from the crown chakra, so as not to create too much heat. This practice causes the secretion of a different type of saliva that has a sweet or Soma content to it and further nourishes the body and mind.

In this process, both the crown and root chakras feed each other. The crown chakra Soma is built up by the lunar energy arising from the root chakra below. The root chakra fire is built up by the fiery energy descending from the crown chakra above. *This process is behind many secret Yoga practices. In this way the Kundalini can ascend but without causing excess heat. Before the Kundalini Shakti can ascend, it must gain the fire from the head. Before the Soma nectar can descend, it must gain the water from the lower chakras.* That is why efforts to raise the Kundalini Shakti without the proper preparation often fail or have side effects.

Once this building up the chakras is completed, the Kundalini can fully awaken and begin the radical ascent of her lightning-fire from below, which energizes each of the chakras along the spine, culminating in the full opening of the crown chakra in all of its glory. Once the nectar is prepared in the head and the root fire is awakened, an opposite movement occurs of an ascending fire and descending nectar. *Yet some Yogis can cause the Kundalini to arise through this lunar pranayama alone. In this way the Kundalini can ascend but without causing excess heat. The Kundalini is carried by the coolness of the ascending Moon.*

I have been observing this lunar breath in myself for some years. The Moon ascends from the root to the crown chakra and then eventually descends into the solar force into the heart, which is experienced overall as a kind of expansion. The meditative power of the mind increases along with the sense of Pure Being in the heart. The Agni or fire below is also strengthened by this solar descent.[62] There is a flow of bliss and an expanse of the crown chakra as well.

Soma Mantras

Relative to mantra practice, there are special 'Soma mantras', like the Panchadashi mantra (**Ka E Ī La Hrīṁ, Ha Sa Ka Ha La Hrīṁ, Sa Ka La Hrīṁ**), which help turn the crown chakra into Soma.

Perhaps more important and safer than attempting Kundalini mantras to awaken the Kundalini, is the repetition of Soma mantras to cool and calm the mind. This opening of the crown chakra is the basis of the worship of *Sri Vidya* and the form of the *Sri Chakra*, which symbolizes the crown chakra. The crown chakra is the seat of all mantras represented by the thousand-syllables of its thousand petals. Such crown chakra mantras are different than the pranic fire mantras used to arouse the Kundalini from below and usually have a cooling and lunar energy.

Vedic Soma mantras (such as make up the ninth book of the *Rigveda*) are also important for stimulating the crown chakra. These Vedic mantras are not based on bijas or single syllable sounds, like most Tantric mantras, but on a metrical pattern called *chandas*,[63] according to which the Vedic hymns or *Suktas* are composed. The complex sound pattern of the Vedic verses helps energize the thousand petals of the crown chakra.

Soma Meditation

Meditation is another important method for preparing the elixir of the crown chakra, particularly 'silent meditation' that gently holds the mind in a state of calm, peace, contentment and delight. The mind should be made still and serene like a mountain lake in which the Soma plant or mystic flower can naturally grow. When the mind learns to love stillness, which is its original nature, then the inner nectar begins to develop of its own accord. This requires a deep contemplative flow of awareness within, with our awareness free of all perturbation, agitation and dualistic opinions. Contemplation of the Absolute or the formless Brahman, the serene Godhead beyond time, space and karma, is a good way to do this.

Merging the mind (crown chakra) into the heart is another way of looking at the process of opening the crown chakra. When the mind becomes merged into the heart, it naturally becomes calm and content. This mind or head sunk into the heart is another aspect of the headless or no-mind condition. The heart becomes all and the head loses its separate existence. The heart consumes the mystic nectar, which feeds its light of love and wisdom.

Becoming the Soma

The soul or the human being is the Soma or food for the Gods. To open the crown chakra, we must become an offering ourselves. Preparing this immortal nectar is not a mechanical thing. The nectar is the essence or rasa of all that we do and are. Unless our lives become an offering for the Gods, the nectar will remain in a raw state. The unrefined nectar will eventually become the poison of sorrow if we do not learn the secret of its transmutation.

We are all seeking the Soma or the mystic nectar, just as we are all following our bliss however we may conceive it to be. The real Soma is within us, though hidden behind our senses and minds. Ultimately, we are the Soma and if we offer ourselves to the divinity within us, then bliss will pervade us on every side! Offer all that you are, all that you love and wish to be, to the Divine Self within. Then the Soma will always be with you.

The Spiritual Heart and the Crown Chakra

As Deities of Yoga, Shiva and Shakti reveal many secrets of the internal energies of Yoga practice. Perhaps none of these are more important than the connections between the spiritual heart and the crown chakra, the two main centers of higher awareness.

Shiva in his Vedic form as Rudra relates to the spiritual heart, the seat of the soul and the higher Self. Shakti, on the other hand, in the Vedic form as Soma, relates to the crown chakra, the thousand petal lotus. One can worship Shiva as the spiritual heart, and complementarily honor Shakti as the crown chakra. Shiva is the Chid-Jyoti or light of consciousness, the deepest light of the core of the heart. Shakti is the play of bliss or Ananda, which arises from the opening of the crown chakra.

Shiva is the root and Shakti is the leaves, flowers and fruit, with the heart being the root of the tree and the head being the flowers. Shiva is the pure awareness of the One only, the Self as Brahman in the heart. Shakti is the comprehensive awareness of the all, the Infinite, the 'everything is Brahman' or *Sarvam Khalvidam Brahma*[64] in the head and through the senses.

The unitary pure light of Shiva from the heart becomes reflected into the variegated effulgence of Shakti in the head. Shiva

213

in the heart provides the focus, the cohesion and the core. Shakti in the head provides the expanse, the vastness and the unbounded unknown. It is a single process viewed from two sides, the center of a circle (Shiva) and its periphery (Shakti).

Some of us might feel confused about identifying Shakti with the head, thinking that Shakti is more a matter of feeling than thinking. In this regard, we should recognize that the crown chakra is not the intellect, though it does impart a brilliance and creativity to the mind. The open crown chakra is a state of no mind, in which the ordinary mind and its dualistic constructs are put to rest. It is a Voidness that possesses tremendous creative powers, the dazzling spectrum of the universal Shakti, like the expanse of universal space which contains all the stars and planets. The open crown chakra endows one with superlative powers of speech, mantra, poetry and vision that can make one into a seer or rishi. It grants us inspirations and insights which reflect the deepest intuition, wisdom, love and bliss. The open crown chakra or 'spiritual head' is our God given field of bliss.

Similarly, the spiritual heart is different than the emotional heart, which is a fragmentation of our deeper feeling potential at a personal level. The spiritual heart is a state of pure feeling and direct knowing that transcends ordinary dualistic emotions of love and hate, like and dislike. It provides direct insight, enduring calm and silence, and an ability to go beyond all names, forms and expressions, yet with a deep sense of compassion, love and courage.

Rudra is the heart. He is ruddy or red, the color of blood. He makes us cry, feel pain and sorrow. When he shoots his arrow, he never misses the target. Whenever we move out of the spiritual heart and into the emotional or reactive heart, Rudra's bow is drawn against us. Whenever we move out of the aspirations of the spiritual heart for the desires of the worldly heart, Shiva's grace becomes wrath. We fall into the realm of sorrow or Samsara and its destructive whirlpools.

Actually, we must first drink the cup of the heart, the blood of feeling, before we can drink the cup of Soma, the nectar of immorality in the head. We must drink all the sorrows and suffering of life, giving reverence to the wrath of fierce Rudra before the nectar of Soma can come to us. When the blood of sorrow has been fully drunk, then the Soma will never cease flowing. We must go through the experience of Rudra, the inner purification, the widening of our minds and hearts into the Infinite and Eternal, before Shakti's stream can fill us with delight. This is what the worship of Kali, who is the Shakti of Shiva as Rudra, brings to us as well. We must experience Kali in the heart before we can reach Sundari in the head.

As Shiva and Shakti are one, so are the spiritual heart and the crown chakra. We open the crown chakra when we merge the mind into the heart. Then the mind, like a phoenix, is resurrected out of the fire of the heart as the mind of Soma, the crown chakra and the fountain of bliss.

The problem for us is that the heart and the head ordinarily move in opposite directions, which means that Shiva and Shakti do not meet; a condition that leads to conflict and fragmentation. Unless we reverse this flow and unite the head with the heart, we cannot find unity, peace or happiness, or the union of the God and the Goddess within us.

To merge Shakti into Shiva is to merge the mind into the heart. This is not merely to merge the intellectual mind into the emotional heart but to merge all our thinking, feeling and cognitive processes as instinct, sensation, emotion, reason and imagination into the serene light of the spiritual heart within. When Shakti fully merges into Shiva then there is the complete stillness of the One beyond all duality.

Yet once Shakti is merged into Shiva, a new Shakti arises out of Shiva. The surrendered individual mind arises as the cosmic mind of the crown chakra. From its innumerable facets, its thousand inner windows on the universe, one can discern the secrets of creation, the birth of all the worlds, the endless stream of karma, and the play of all the cosmic essences (rasas and tanmatras) from the infinitesimal to the infinite. Looking at the world through the crown chakra, every form is a doorway to infinity and every event is a gateway to eternity. The crown chakra expands endlessly in all directions. It is an unlimited explosion of Shakti as a perpetual radiance of lightning in all possible dimensions.

When Shiva enters into Shakti—that is when the spiritual heart awareness looks through the crown chakra—the full expansiveness of Brahman is revealed, in which all the universes are but waves and bubbles on an infinite sea. And yet each object also becomes as vast and infinite as Brahman. One is in all and all is in one's Self that has no limits.

When Shakti enters into Shiva—that is when the crown chakra is merged in the spiritual heart—then all creation dissolves back into the depths of the heart, where there is no other, no object, no time or space, not even the possibility or the conception of anything. Even the distinction of Shiva and Shakti disappears. This interweaving of Shiva and Shakti as the spiritual heart and the crown chakra is the bliss of Self-realization.

The Chakras
and the Spiritual Heart

Most Tantric Yoga approaches emphasize the seven chakras, with the highest Self-realization occurring with the opening of the crown chakra or thousand petal lotus of the head. However, the Yoga of Knowledge and many ancient teachings like the *Upanishads* and the *Bhagavad Gita* emphasizes the heart instead, as in this Upanishadic statement.

> *As far as space extends, so far is this space within the heart. Placed in it are both Heaven and Earth, in it are both Fire and Wind (Agni and Vayu), both Sun and Moon (Surya and Chandra), both Lightning and the stars, whatever is here and whatever is not here, all of that is placed within the heart.*
> —*Chandogya Upanishad VIII.3*

The *Yoga Sutras* III.33 similarly regards the origin of the mind or chitta to be in the heart. "Through meditation on the heart, comes knowledge of the chitta."

The *hridaya* or spiritual heart is said to be the place where the Atman or higher Self dwells. The teachings of Ramana Maharshi, perhaps the greatest enlightened sage of modern India, center on bringing one's awareness back to the heart, from which there is no ascent or descent, no coming and going. Those more familiar with the idea of the seven chakras may be confused by this. Is not the heart chakra only a halfway point in the process?

The spiritual heart (hridaya) is not the same as the heart chakra, which is called *Anahata* in Sanskrit, though it does have a close connection with it. The spiritual heart is not simply a place on the spine or an energy center in the subtle body. It is the core of awareness that is both the basis of the causal body (the seat of the reincarnating soul) and the Supreme Self beyond all manifestation. It contains all the chakras and yet is beyond them.

To understand the movement of Yoga at a deeper level, it is important to understand the following principle: *All the chakras open to merge back into the crown chakra, which in turn opens to merge back into the spiritual heart.* The inner Yoga is a single process of the expansion of awareness happening in different rhythms and dimensions. *The different chakras, starting with the root chakra, are aspects of the crown chakra, which in turn is contained in the spiritual heart.*

We can identify the spiritual heart with the Sushumna or spinal nadi itself. Ascending the Sushumna is also a process of opening the spiritual heart. The Kundalini Shakti is not just a movement up the Sushumna but an expansion of awareness in the Sushumna itself, an expansion of the spiritual heart. The Sushumna in itself is experienced as space or the Void. One need not actually move out of the Sushumna into the different chakras but can remain in it, going directly to the crown chakra and the spiritual heart.

The crown chakra contains the other six chakras within itself. The vertical ascent and opening of the chakras can also be viewed on a horizontal plane as different stages of the opening the crown chakra itself. Similarly, the spiritual heart is the essence of the crown chakra, its deepest core, with the crown chakra being its outer expansion.

All deities, all worlds and all creatures exist in the spiritual heart, where one's true Self dwells as the root of the mind, prana and speech. In the heart is the ultimate essence of Soma or the mystic nectar, and of Agni, the sacred fire, as well as the inner Sun and the inner Moon. Shiva and Shakti are the two sides of the spiritual heart as its immutable peace (Shiva) and its infinite expansion (Shakti).

To understand these subtle variations, remember that inner Yoga practice deals with formless energies and states of awareness, not with fixed objects in the physical world that can be precisely defined in time-space terms. Yoga requires that we understand the logic of the infinite and the universal, which is a movement of inner integration, not a creation of rigid outer distinctions.

One is always in the spiritual heart, which is the root of all states of consciousness. Any ascent or descent of consciousness must occur within it. Yet there are certain energetics involved in yogic processes, which various practitioners will experience differently. These can be felt subjectively in a vivid way as an ascent or descent, a movement within, an expansion or a centering, with alternating rhythms and flows.

The movement of the Kundalini fire up the spine is complemented by a descending flow of nectar, amrit, Soma or grace, while an expansion occurs at the level of the heart as the unfoldment of a solar force. The different ways how these forces move is important for particular Yoga practices, even though ultimately, as part of the same process of Self-realization, they dissolve into the One and their details are forgotten.

The development of the Kundalini is but one angle, though very important, of viewing how the energy of consciousness develops. We can look at it in other ways like the expansion of the Divine Word **OM**, as a sharpening of the concentration power of the one-pointed mind, as the friction of Self-inquiry, or as the passion of devotion. One should not put much emphasis on any name but be able to recognize the underlying factors, which must be present in all yogic realization as a deep samadhi or absorption within.

Just as the spiritual heart is the seat of the Divine Self, the supreme Deity, the chakras are the centers of various deities that rule over the elements, senses, qualities and energies of the chakras. Entering into the chakras, the Shakti energy takes the form of various Goddesses, which can appear blissful or terrifying depending upon one's inner condition. Yet if one surrenders to the Goddess, she will also return us to the spiritual heart, opening up all the other chakras along the way as a blossoming of her abundance.

The bija mantra **Hrīm**, the *Devi Pranava* or 'seed-syllable of the Goddess', is also the mantra of the hridaya or spiritual heart. Through it we can enter into the small space or cavern within the heart, in which all the universe is contained. Alternatively, we can use her three heart mantras for this purpose:

Hrīm Śrīm Klīm

Hrīm is the energy of the heart. **Śrīm** is the devotion of the heart. **Klīm** is the love and wishes of the heart. Or we can use the fifteen syllable Panchadashi Mantra, which is the extended form of **Hrīm**, adding **Hrīm** to the beginning as the sixteenth factor:

Hrīm, Ka E Ī La Hrīm, Ha Sa Ka Ha La Hrīm, Sa Ka La Hrīm

We should consecrate our entire being—body, speech, breath, mind and heart—into the inner Divinity that is our real identity. Then we will return to the supreme abode in which abides the unity of Shiva and Shakti and of all dualities. This is our natural state of pure existence, when we give up the distractions of the outer world.

May you return to your inner heart, your inner home in the bosom of the Infinite Mother and the Eternal Father. May you discover your true Self and manifest its universal peace for the benefit of all! May you experience all the chakras, all the worlds and all beings as woven on the grace of the heart and as expressions of your own deepest nature!

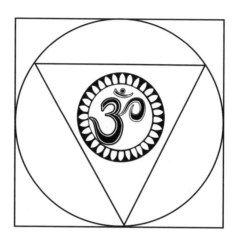

Atma-Shakti,
The Power of the Self

The universe is a marvelous, awesome, and unpredictable effulgence of power or Shakti. It is an ongoing cataclysmic event of incredible transformations at multiple levels and many dimensions from the subatomic to the supragalactic. Yet this display of universal power is rooted in an equally vast consciousness. If we do not recognize that universal consciousness, we may experience the beauty and marvels of nature but we will remain ignorant of the real meaning of it all!

The cosmic energy or Shakti is a force of awareness, beauty and delight, not a mere material or unconscious power. However, it is a force of consciousness beyond the human mind, whose logic transcends the limited patterns of our human rationality. Shakti reflects the working of an all pervasive intelligence, not circumscribed by the needs of any creaturely mind. It acts for the unfoldment of universal potentials, not merely for the benefit of a particular individual or group.

This universal power is the inner current that endows us with life, love and wisdom. It is the steady and determined force behind the beating of our hearts. It is the continuous rhythmic dance behind the movement of our breath. It is the subtle mental energy behind the arising of all the thoughts within us from birth to death.

Ultimately, this energy of existence is the very power of the Self or *Atma-Shakti*. This power of the Self gives rise to all other powers. It is from our sense of Self or 'I am' that all our other senses arise and through which they are able to function. It is from our sense of self that we gain energy, prana and motivation for all our actions. It is from this 'I' throbbing within us that our hearts can beat and our minds can think. Its force arises impetuously and imperiously at every moment behind all that we do and attempt. No one can stop it without ceasing to be.

The *Upanishads* speak of the *Devatma Shakti*, the 'power of the Divine Self', that gets hidden in the qualities of nature as it moves into manifestation.[65] This is the supreme power that we must recognize in order to find any real peace or happiness, not the sanction of any external deity or human leader.

The problem is that we have forgotten the Self-power within us and instead run after the forces of the external world, seeking recognition or support from the outside. We lose our own inner strength and confidence and come under the domination of other people. In this process, a spiritual entropy occurs, resulting in fragmentation and sorrow.

Yet if we can but turn our energies within, we will discover this universal Self-power as the real energy behind life and regain our true dignity, awareness and freedom. For this to occur, we must reclaim our spiritual independence, which is to become our own center of original awareness and insight, not simply a product of our education, environment or the media influences around us.

To reclaim our inner strength, we must learn to merge all our energies into the Self-power within. We can do this by directing the energy of our prana, senses, mind and emotions back to the root power of the heart within, the 'mantric beating of the spiritual heart' that occurs behind the physical heart. The spiritual heart of pure awareness is always beating as 'I am all', which is the source of real vitality and joy in all creatures.

The Self is Shiva in its state of rest and Shakti in its state of motion. Awakened Shakti, the inner power of Yoga, naturally takes us back to the Self. It leads us to the energy behind the form and the consciousness behind the energy. We must awaken this *Atma-Shakti* or 'Self-power' in order to integrate and internalize all other Shaktis. The Atma-Shakti is the Mother Shakti behind all the Goddesses and all the Gods.

All the chakras dwell in the spiritual heart which in its highest level is the seat of the Self, the Atman within. Balance and awaken all the energies within yourself by coming into contact with your real Self beyond body and mind, time and space. Merge your speech, mind and prana into it as their true origin at the core of your being.

Look at the energies of your body and mind, as well as those of the external world, as forms of Shakti rooted in the Atma-Shakti, the Self-power that is the supreme Devata. Trace the root of all energies to their source within your own inner being and deeper consciousness. Then your energy will resonate with the energy of the entire universe as the play of Shiva and Shakti.

Our bodies are manifestations of intelligence and consciousness, vehicles of expression and action for the inner soul. The entire universe is a meditative display of wonder and delight originating from the highest awareness. Even the power of the wind reflects the presence of the formless spirit and is not simply an unconscious force. We must learn to reclaim all energy in the universe as our own, with the entire universe as the exuberance of our own immortal vitality.

This 'spiritualization of energy' is the best way to get beyond any energy crisis and to become free of all external energy needs. When our life merges into the universal energy, then everything

becomes a miraculous event without any change of appearance!
Every day becomes an effulgence of the highest Shakti!

Contact your own Self-power, not as a limited self-assertion
but as the universality of awareness. Reclaim all the powers of the
universe as your own vitality, just as the entire universe is your
home, resting contentedly in your inner Self that is connected to
all that is or all that ever could be.

APPENDIX ONE

Teachings and Tradition

This section will examine the intellectual, cultural and historical ramifications of the Inner Yoga, both Tantric and Vedic, drawing correlations, including keys to help the student connect to the deeper and broader traditions.

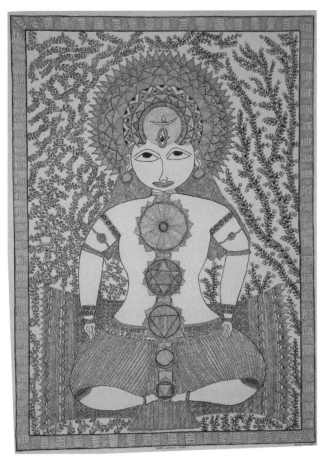

The Question of Tradition

The Yoga tradition reflects a radically different view of humanity than our current civilization. In Vedic thought, which classical Yoga is part of, true knowledge is inherent in the Cosmic Mind or *Mahat Tattva* in the Yoga system. Individuals can raise their awareness to access such universal knowledge, but it not the invention or possession of any person or group. A higher yogic knowledge has always been present in humanity. Such spiritual knowledge was in fact more common in ancient times and earlier yugas (world-ages) before the human mind had descended into materialism (the dark age of Kali Yuga).

Our current science and technology is the result of outgoing or rajasic tendencies that do not reflect our highest urges as a species. Our current accounts of history and civilization based upon this materialistic view of humanity are flawed by yogic standards. They miss the real essence of human striving, which is the pursuit of Self-realization, not simply political, economic or technological development. This distorted historical vision has colored how we view Yoga, Tantra and Veda, which is usually to separate them into warring camps as conflicting belief systems.

Yoga rests upon a great tradition, said to go back to the very origins of human culture before what we regard of as history began, called the 'Eternal Dharma' or *Sanatana Dharma* in Sanskrit. Understanding this tradition is not a mere academic matter but goes to the core of what Yoga is all about. The Yoga tradition has developed and carries a special body of inner knowledge. We could compare the experiential tradition of Yoga with that of science. Just as a scientist today cannot ignore the greater tradition of science and go far in his research, so too a real yogi cannot ignore the greater tradition of Yoga and go very far in his practice. Teachings that have been practiced by great yogis for centuries gain a special power and efficacy that a mere individual today cannot create. Traditions provide *samskaras* or 'seed energies' that support the individual and allow us to accomplish what we could never achieve on our own.

However, few Yoga practitioners today understand the greater tradition of Yoga. They often look at Yoga according to the views of academics and scholars who are outside the Yoga tradition, if not opposed to it. Such non-yogic views on Yoga breed many misunderstandings that prevent people from reaching the deeper practices of the inner Yoga and keep them caught in the outer Yoga of asana only.

Tradition is also important in Yoga as 'lineage', a living connection with guru lines, the *guru-sishya parampara*. A Yoga lineage provides a human link to the tradition and its various branches. To become part of the Yoga tradition is not just an outer formality of joining one group or another, but the ability to connect to great teachers and teachings at a heart level. Great gurus have created inner paths that we can follow, just as previous generations have created roads that we can drive on. There is an 'inner tradition' that we can access within ourselves if we gain the right receptivity.

Perhaps more importantly, a real yogic tradition connects us to the Devatas, the great Gods and Goddesses that sustain the higher teachings in the Cosmic Mind. There are Divine forces behind an authentic tradition we can connect to in a transformative manner, like linking to a power source. For Devata or Deity Yoga in particular, the tradition carries not only the living connection to the guru but also to the Deity.

The classical Yoga tradition as part of *Sanatana Dharma* is related to all Vedic and sacred sciences like Ayurveda, Vedic astrology and Vastu. No sect or lineage in the Yoga tradition exists apart from these broader teachings. Without a recognition of this greater Vedic tradition that classical Yoga is part of, students can end up with narrow views, regarding their guru, lineage or approach as the only authentic one. It is important for serious students to study the greater tradition, or their ability to apply their particular lineages may be limited.

Note that I have examined the issues of ancient history directly in a number of other publications, including the Vedic nature of the ancient civilization of India.[66] Much new literature on this subject has come out from many important authors.[67] It is enough here to say that the Yoga tradition sees a continual tradition in India from Vedic to Puranic and Tantric lines. This is a view that great modern gurus like Vivekananda, Aurobindo and Yogananda have already mentioned. Though names and forms have changed, the essence of the tradition, its teachings and practices remains the same.

Tantra and Non-duality

Misconceptions about Tantra are common relative to Tantric philosophy as well. In this regard, many scholars view Tantric philosophy as fundamentally different from Vedantic philosophies of world negation (what is called *Mayavada* in Sanskrit), which reject the universe as an illusion only, while Tantra affirms the world as real. They contrast Tantra with non-dualistic (Advaita) Vedantic schools, as if the two were very far apart. They exaggerate minor differences and miss deeper and more profound connections.

Certainly differences do exist between Advaita Vedanta and Tantric philosophies, but these are no more than those that exist between different Vedantic or Tantric philosophies in or among themselves. Most importantly, Tantra itself, in all of its variations, is a Vedantic school in the broader sense of the term, in that its philosophy uses a Vedantic terminology of Self (Atman), God (Ishvara) and the Absolute (Brahman) and its practices are similar types of rituals, mantras, pranayamas and meditations.

Tantra, like Yoga and Vedanta, has as its highest goal the realization of the underlying unity of all existence, the Self or Brahman. The term Tantra itself refers to the 'connecting thread', the unity that runs through everything, which is a unity of Shiva and Shakti, light and energy, awareness and bliss. To discover the real truth of Tantra is to work with the forces of duality in order to go beyond duality.

Tantra reduces the great multiplicity of forces in the universe to the two primal powers of Shiva and Shakti in order to merge these two into One Brahman. After all, the closest number to one is the number two. The polarity of duality rests upon the energy of unity. The attraction of opposites, through which all energy is created, is the attraction of a deeper unity to which they long to return.

Tantra does have its mundane side—as do Vedic and Puranic teachings—which addresses the outer needs of people relative to health, happiness and prosperity. Traditional Tantra, like the

Veda, contains teachings for all levels of individuals and all the main goals of life. Tantra is like a great mother who provides food and guidance for all her children, even those who may be spiritually immature.

There are Tantric teachings for gaining relationship partners, for sexual enjoyment, for having good children, gaining wealth or even for the defeat of enemies. There are also Vedic rituals and mantras that can be used for such worldly ends. Such mundane Tantra does not necessarily put Veda and Tantra overall at odds as some scholars would like to believe, but we do need to discriminate between lower and higher sides of teachings, whether Tantric or Vedic.

The practices of Tantra can be abused or misapplied for selfish ends, to control, dominate or even harm—though this will eventually backfire on those who do this and leave them in pain or confusion. There is a dark Tantra that uses lesser deities, mantras and even ghosts for such destructive ends. Though this is a subject of much fascination for people like the sexual side of Tantra, it is only the shadow of the deeper spiritual Tantra.

Tantric philosophies are of several types, and recognize various levels of teachings relative to the maturity or ripeness of the disciple. Yet most Tantric philosophies are ultimately non-dualistic (unitarian) in nature and affirm the oneness of the individual soul or Jivatman with the Supreme Self or Paramatman. *And there is a Tantric school inherent in Advaita or non-dualistic Vedanta itself.*

The greatest of all the Advaitic gurus, Shankara, wrote important Tantric works and performed Tantric Yoga practices. Shankara's long poem, *Saundarya Lahari*, the 'Wave of Bliss', remains one of the most important of all Tantric teachings. It dominates the Tantric tradition of the South of India, whose overall system of Agamic temple worship is Tantric in nature as well. *Saundarya Lahari* provides the keys to the worship of the Goddess in terms of forms, mantras and yantras up to the details of the highest Sri Vidya, the worship of Sri Chakra. This tradition has continued throughout the Advaitic Swami orders in India. All the main Shankara Maths or monastic centers in India have various Devis installed who are worshiped regularly with Tantric mantras and rituals.

Many traditional Tantric texts like the *Devi Bhagavata Purana,* in which the famous *Devi Mahatymam* (Chandi Path) occurs, or the *Shiva Gita* from the *Padma Purana*, are Advaitic in philosophy, following a similar line to Shankara and teach the absolute unity of the Self and Brahman. Generally, most texts that emphasize the worship of the Goddess or Devi are non-dualistic in orientation, whereas those to Vishnu are dualistic, and only some of those to Shiva are non-dualistic.

The Kashmiri Shaivite system—such as expressed in the teachings of the great guru Abhinavagupta—is probably the most dominant and comprehensive of the Tantric systems of philosophy. Its approach is also Advaitic or non-dualistic, though with slight differences from the teachings of Shankara. The Kashmir Shaivite system grants a more positive reality to the world as a meditative expression of pure consciousness (which some have argued is the original view of the *Upanishads* and older Vedanta), but it hardly regards the world as real in a modern materialistic or scientific sense. Apart from a few such technical points, its teaching and practices are essentially the same as that of Shankara, extolling Self-realization and similar means to attain it through Self-inquiry, mantra, Yoga and meditation. Therefore, one need not make too much of the differences between these two non-dualistic systems (Advaita Vedanta and Kashmiri Shaivism), which are both part of the same greater tradition.

Many great modern non-dualist Vedantins have been Devi worshippers and used Tantric Yoga methods as well. We see this with Paramahansa Ramakrishna, who was a devotee of Kali. Sri Aurobindo, Paramahansa Yogananda and Swami Shivananda of Rishikesh worshipped the Goddess as well as accepted the philosophy of Vedanta at a non-dualistic level (though Aurobindo developed his own system apart from that of Shankara). In addition, many of the great women gurus of modern India, like Sharada Devi, the wife of Ramakrishna, Anandamayi Ma and Ammachi, whose disciples often worship them as the Goddess, have taught the non-dualistic approach of Vedanta.

Ramana Maharshi, the greatest of the modern Advaitic gurus of modern India, included Devi worship in his ashram rituals. Worship of the Sri Yantra is done regularly at the Ramanashram even today. Ganapati Muni, the chief disciple of Ramana, was himself a great Devi worshiper who helped formally institute these practices at the ashram. The teachings of the current book are based on Ganapati Muni's work and follow his view of the unity of Veda, Tantra and Yoga.

Devi worship has been an integral part of Advaita Vedanta in India from ancient times to modern masters. However, it follows the *Dakshinachara* or 'right-handed path' of Tantra, emphasizing Self-realization as the goal. Followers of the 'left-handed path' or *Vamachara* are more likely to have a dualistic view of reality. In addition, though Tantrics may accept Non-duality at a philosophical level, their practices can be different than ascetic Yoga approaches, and may emphasize a more positive use of the senses, emotions and body, and a greater receptivity to the forces of nature.

In any case, the differences between Tantra and Vedanta as dualistic and non-dualistic cover much of the same ground as between the different Vedantic traditions as dualistic or non-dualistic, with the followers of devotion or Bhakti Yoga preferring a view of duality and those of knowledge of Jnana Yoga preferring non-duality.

Shakti and the Vedas

A number of scholars and writers have tried to divide the two great traditions of India, Veda and Tantra, as different or contrary. A few Indian Yoga teachers have uncritically taken up this view as well, though the great majority like Vivekananda, Aurobindo and Yogananda have not accepted it. Such scholars usually identify the Vedic tradition with proposed invading Aryans from Central Asia and the Tantric tradition with indigenous Dravidians.

However, now the Aryan Invasion theory is severely in question, having failed to produce any archaeological or genetic data to prove itself. No such invading Aryans or their artifacts have ever been found. Meanwhile, the Sarasvati River of Vedic fame, which once flowed between the Indus and the Ganga, has been found to be the main homeland of civilization in ancient India before it finally dried up around 2000 BCE. In light of this new information, we should reexamine the connections between Veda and Tantra as well.

Vedic and Tantric traditions are one, though with different orientations and nomenclature. The Vedic tradition is an earlier form of the Tantric, which itself is a later development of certain Vedic practices. Tantric teachings abound in rituals and mantras connected to the Vedic. Most notably, inner Tantric Yoga reflects the four main Vedic deities of Agni, Soma, Vayu and Surya (the forces of fire, moon, wind and sun) as the main forces of the psyche.

Perhaps the easiest correlation to bear in mind is that the *Vedas* emphasize the *Jyotirmaya Purusha*, 'the Being or Person made of light', while the *Tantras* emphasize the *Shaktimaya Devi*, 'the Goddess made of energy'. Yet light and energy as consciousness and force are one. The Purusha of light is one with its energy or Shakti. *We could call the Vedic Yoga a 'Vedic Light Yoga' and the Tantric Yoga a 'Tantric Energy Yoga'*. The two are not only related historically but are complementary in their mantras and practices and have commonly been used together.

The Vedic view emphasizes the Shiva principle, though under the abstract forms of Brahman, Purusha and Atman, and as different Vedic deities (like Agni and Soma), which reflect the cosmic masculine energy and light form identified with Shiva. Yet the *Vedas* also recognize the Shakti principle as *Vak* or the power of the Divine Word, which is said to be *Veda-Mata* or 'Mother of the *Vedas*'. The Goddess pervades the *Vedas*, not so much as a particular deity but as the Vedic mantra itself! This includes the Vedic meters like Gayatri, which are all regarded as feminine in nature.

The Tantric view emphasizes the Shakti principle as the great Goddess but recognizes the light principle with Shiva as Prakasha or pure illumination. It also aims at the realization of Atman and Brahman, defined both as the light and energy of consciousness, Chid-Jyoti and Chit-Shakti.

Another difference between Vedic and Tantric Yogas is that the Vedic deities are primarily powers of nature like Fire, Wind, Sun and Moon. Their anthropomorphic sides are secondary and seldom clearly delineated. Agni, for example, is primarily the deity of fire. Though he is at times presented as a human child or as a young man, this is only one aspect of his many forms in nature. Tantric Deities like Shiva and Shakti, on the other hand, have a more vivid anthropomorphic symbolism as the Divine Father and Mother, to which their nature forms are usually subordinated. Of course, this distinction is just one of degree as naturalistic and anthropomorphic sides exist to both Vedic and Tantric symbolisms.

The *Vedas* center on the four great Devatas or principles of light in the universe as Agni (Fire), Soma (Moon), Indra-Vayu (Lightning) and Surya (Sun). Yet each of these forms of light has its corresponding forms of energy as fire energy, lunar energy, solar energy and electrical energy.

Tantric Yoga uses these same forces as Sun, Moon, Lightning and Fire as Goddesses. Soma, the lunar reflective force, is the

Goddess Lalita or Tripura Sundari and the crown chakra. Indra relates to Tantric Chinnamasta as the power of lightning perception in the eyes. Surya is the solar power of life and awareness in the heart, which is Bhadra Kali among the Goddesses. Agni is the Kundalini fire in the root chakra, which is Bhairavi. Vayu is the general Kriya Shakti force that is Kali in the broader sense.

Both Vedic and Tantric Yogas revolve around awakening these four light and energy centers in the body: the Fire in the three lower chakras, the Moon in the three higher chakras, and the Sun in the heart, with Lightning in the third eye. The Tantric Shiva-Shakti Yoga is another form of the Vedic Agni-Soma ritual on an internal level. Tantric Yoga, which aims balancing Agni and Soma, is a development of the Vedic Yoga. This is by way of summary of what we have discussed already in the book.

On a practical level, there are also no major differences between Veda and Tantra. Each teaches various levels of practices from the mundane to the transcendent. Even the Vamachara or 'the left-handed path of Tantra', which is often regarded as non-Vedic, has a counterpart in certain Vedic rituals involving a ritual usage of intoxicants, meat or sexual practices.[68] Yet for both Tantra and Veda, the right-handed Dakshinachara approach, which emphasizes sattvic values like the yamas and niyamas of classical Yoga, has usually been emphasized as the highest. What is usually criticized as unspiritual is the Vamachara, not the deeper or inner Tantric Yoga.

Shakti and the *Vedas*

The Vedic rishis honored Shakti primarily as *Vak* or the 'power of the Divine Word'. Vedic mantras are the manifestations of the Shakti of Divine Speech, carrying the power of all creation and the secrets of cosmogenesis. The *Rig-Veda* itself is a creation of Kundalini Shakti, which is the power of Vak or Divine Speech, as it manifested at the beginning of this particular Yuga or World-age, not merely in individuals but in great families of seers or Rishis. *The Rig-Veda itself is perhaps the greatest mantric effusion of Kundalini Shakti at a collective level that has ever occurred.*

The Shakti of the Vedic hymns is the strongest of all Sanskrit hymns, their many syllables reflecting the rhythms of cosmic creation and the thousand syllables of the crown chakra. However, bija mantras like **Hrīm** and **Śrīm** are more defined in Tantra, though they are hidden in the roots of Vedic words,[69] and do occur in Vedic and Upanishadic teachings.[70] Tantric bijas are the strongest of all bijas, the primal sounds behind the universe. One could say that the *Vedas* reflect the metrical power of Sanskrit, whereas Tantra reflects its seed sounds. Sanskrit meanwhile is no mere human dialect but a human emulation of the vibratory patterns underlying the very laws and energies of the greater universe. That is why it has such a power to change our consciousness. No other language can compare to it in this respect.

Tantric Yoga follows a Vedic approach connecting the creation of the universe with the development of the Sanskrit alphabet starting with *OM*. Kashmir Shaivism contains an elaborate system of relating the letters of the Sanskrit alphabet to all the cosmic principles from the Absolute to the earth element. It views the Sanskrit letters as the Shaktis and the Mothers (Matrikas) through which everything in the universe is energized.[71]

The older Vedic tradition contains a similar emphasis on the Sanskrit alphabet and letters, though many of the details have been lost. According the *Upanishads*,[72] the vowels relate to Indra as the supreme deity, just as they do to Shiva in the Tantric tradition. In the *Aitareya Aranyaka*, an even older Vedic text, the letter-*a* is said to be the Brahman,[73] and the sibilants or *s* and *h* sounds are said to relate to Prana, just as in later Tantra.[74] The great system of Kashmir Shaivism with its deities, mantras, pranas and tattvas reflecting the Sanskrit alphabet is another formulation of the older Vedic model. In fact, *it is in the Tantric Mantra Yoga that we find the continuation of the Vedic Mantra Yoga that was the main Vedic Yoga.*

Shiva and the *Vedas*

Shiva, if we look deeply, is the Supreme Deity of the Rig-Veda and its four main light forms as Agni (Fire), Soma (Moon), Surya (Sun) and Indra (Lightning). This statement may seem unusual, if not absurd, for those used to thinking that *Vedas* and *Agamas* are different or that Shiva is not a Vedic deity, because his particular name and form is not much present there. The problem is that such views are only looking superficially at the names not to the inner meaning.

Shiva is said to be *Agni-Somatmakam*, meaning that he has the 'nature of both Agni and Soma' as fire and water and all the other dualities that they represent. Agni is his fierce or Rudra form. Soma is his blissful form. Shiva is also Surya or the Sun as pure light, Prakasha. As Prana, he is also Vayu, the Lord of the cosmic wind. He is Indra as the lord of perception and the power of mantra. Shiva is the background deity of the Rig-Veda of which the other four main deities are outer forms. These four main Vedic deities can be seen as facets of Shiva or his sons, just as his son Skanda represents Agni or Fire.[75]

Tantric Yoga is the Vedic Yajna internalized; a worship of the inner fire of the Kundalini with pranayama, mantra and meditation. The worship of Shiva also maintains many Vedic forms, using the Vedic fire, Vedic mantras and a Vedic like communion with nature. Shaivite Yogis are famous for their sacred fires, with which they worship with Vedic mantras, anointing their bodies with its ashes. The *Rudram*, the most famous chant to Shiva, which is found in the *Yajur-Veda*, makes Shiva's identity with the Vedic sacrifice very clear.

Veda and Tantra are part of the same greater Yoga tradition that has continued in India since the most ancient times. The names and forms have naturally changed over time but the basic principles and practices have remained the same. Any differences between Vedic and Tantric teachings are within this same greater tradition. All serious Yoga students can benefit by Vedic and Tantric practices and by the Vedantic philosophy that is the essence of both.

APPENDIX TWO

Reference Material

This section includes important information on the pronunciation and chanting mantras, as well as basic reference material for the book as a whole.

I. Note on the Use of Mantras

If you wish to use any of the mantras in the book, please make sure to keep the following factors in mind. Such mantras should be done with care, devotion, a calm mind and steady heart.

1. Chant the mantra only with a sattvic or pure mindset, which means a sattvic or peaceful intention and a calm frame of mind. This means that one should do the mantra only for spiritual purposes and not for personal gain or to harm others. Follow a sattvic or pure life-style while doing the mantra. This includes a vegetarian diet, refraining from negative emotions, time in solitude, and making one's life into a form of service.

2. Honor the deity that is connected to the mantra, whether through mental acknowledgment, some form of ritual, or a representative form like a statue or picture before starting your practice. See the mantra as a manifestation of the deity, not as an inert force to be manipulated. In addition, meditate upon the deity while repeating the mantra.

3. Seek greater teachings about the mantra from gurus, traditions or authoritative texts. Seek further empowerment with the mantra with a guru, a holy site connected to its deity, or through the forces of nature like fire or water.

4. Be careful using harsh or strong mantras like those of Kali or Bhairavi. Balance these with soft or benefic mantras like those of Sundari or Lakshmi. Generally, it is best to start off with the mantra **Hrīm** for the Goddess in all her forms before moving on to other mantras.

5. Make sure to pronounce the mantra properly. For this you may need to learn some of the basic rules of pronunciation of the Sanskrit alphabet, starting with the Sanskrit pronunciation key in the book.

6. Initially chant the mantra out loud to get a sense of its sound pattern. Chant it softly on the breath to connect it to the Prana. But most chanting will be mental or in the mind while one is silent.

7. Chant the mantra in a regular manner at a certain time of day for a certain number of times. Generally single syllable bija mantras like **Krīm** or **Hrīm** require at least 100,000 repetitions to energize, while longer syllable or extended mantras require at least 10,000, done in a series of regular sessions every day or at least once a week for a period of at least one month. More repetition is generally better than less as far as mantra practice goes. Best is to let the mantra repeat itself continually and spontaneously in your subconscious mind. That is a good sign you have really connected to the power of the mantra.

8. For counting mantras, it is best to use a *mala* or rosary of 108 beads. For single syllable bija mantras you can count 8, 16 or 32 repetitions of the mantra per bead to make it easier. 60 rounds are necessary for 100,000 repetitions at 16 per bead, 30 rounds at 32 per bead. For longer mantras, you can count one recitation of the mantra per bead. Chanting the mantra in a fast mode helps energize the Prana. Chanting it slowly helps calm the mind.

9. Once the mantra has been energized, you can repeat at will or follow its movement as it naturally arises within you. You need not continue to count it, though this can still be helpful.

10. Some Tantrics, particularly in India, like to use harsh mantras or deities to control or harm others. This has bad karmic consequences and increases the qualities of rajas and tamas in one's own nature. This is to be entirely avoided. Use mantras for the Inner Yoga only.

2. Phonetic Pronunciation of Mantras

Ām—Ahm

Aim—Aym

Aum—Aum

Dūm—Doom

Ham Saḥ—Hum saha

Haum—Haum

Hrīm—Hreem

Hsklrīṁ—Hsklreem

Hsraiṁ—Hsraym

Hsrauṁ—Hsraum

Hūm—Hoom

Klīm—Kleem

Īm—Eem

Krīm—Kreem

Jūm—Joom

Namaḥ—Namah

OM—Om

Saḥ—Saha

Sauḥ—Sauha

Śrīm—Shreem

So'ham—So hum

Svāhā—Swaha

This table is phonetic, for an easy initial examination of the sounds. For more detail see the Sanskrit pronunciation key.

The m-sound at the end of most bija mantras represents a nasalization of the vowel followed by a closing of the lips, a sound called 'anusvara' in Sanskrit. One should draw the energy of the mantra into the mind through the practice of this special sound.

Note that the a-vowel, without a line on top of it, is always pronounced short as in 'a book' or the word 'the'. The most common mispronunciation of Sanskrit is in making that sound long or different. The same sound is used for naming letters in Sanskrit, which is a language of syllables. For example, the mantras for the elements, **Lam, Vam, Ram, Yam,** and **Ham,** use this short a-sound.

Sanskrit Pronunciation Key

16 Vowels (some have 2 forms)

अ	a	another
आ ा	ā	father (2 beats)
इ ि	i	pin
ई ी	ī	need (2 beats)
उ ु	u	flute
ऊ ू	ū	mood (2 beats)
ऋ ृ	ṛ	macabre
ॠ ॄ	ṝ	trill for 2 beats
ऌ ॢ	ḷr	table
ए े	e	etude (2 beats)
ऐ ै	ai	aisle (2 beats)
ओ ो	o	yoke (2 beats)
औ ौ	au	flautist (2 beats)
अं	aṃ	hum
अः	aḥ	out-breath

Eight Intermediate Sounds

य	ya	employable
र	ra	abra cadabra
ल	la	hula
व	va	variety
श	śa	shut
ष	ṣa	shnapps
स	sa	Lisa
ह	ha	honey

25 Consonants

क	ka	paprika
ख	kha	thick honey
ग	ga	saga
घ	gha	big honey
ङ	ṅa	ink
च	ca	chutney
छ	cha	much honey
ज	ja	Japan
झ	jha	raj honey
ञ	ña	inch
ट	ṭa	borscht again
ठ	ṭha	borscht honey
ड	ḍa	shdum
ढ	ḍha	shd hum
ण	ṇa	shnum
त	ta	pasta
थ	tha	eat honey
द	da	soda
ध	dha	good honey
न	na	banana
प	pa	paternal
फ	pha	scoop honey
ब	ba	scuba
भ	bha	rub honey
म	ma	aroma

Glossary of Sanskrit Terms

Advaita—non-duality

Agni—fire as cosmic, yogic and biological principle

Akarshana Shakti—cosmic attractive force

Akasha—space as cosmic reality

Antar Yoga—Inner Yoga

Antaranga Yoga—Yoga of the inner limbs or aspects of practice

Atman—higher or true Self

Ayurveda—Vedic medicine

Bahiranga Yoga—Yoga of the outer limbs or aspects of practice

Bhairavi—Goddess of fire, specifically Kundalini fire in the root
    chakra

Bhakti—devotion

Bija mantra—seed syllable mantra like **Om** or **Hrīm**

Brahma—creative aspect of Divinity among the trinity

Brahman—the Godhead or Absolute

Buddhi—higher or discriminating aspect of intelligence

Chakra—energy channel of the subtle body

Chitta—the mental field

Chinnamasta—literally 'a cut off head', Goddess governing the
    third eye; also called Vajra Yogini and Prachanda Chandi

Dakinis—Shaktis of the chakras

Deva—Divine being or being of light

Devata—Divine or cosmic principle, deity, God or Goddess

Devi—Goddess

Dharana—concentration as a limb of Yoga practice

Doshas—biological humors of Ayurveda

Drishti Yoga—Yoga of perception

Ganesha—Deity of knowledge, teaching and skill; portrayed
    with the head of an elephant

Hridaya—the spiritual heart and seat of the soul and Self

Indra—Vedic deity governing perception

Ishta Devata—chosen deity for worship

Ishvara—Cosmic Lord or God in theistic sense

Guna—quality of nature, especially three gunas of Sattva, Rajas and Tamas

Jnana—spiritual knowledge

Jyotish—Vedic astrology as science of light

Kala—time as a cosmic reality

Kali—Supreme Goddess as the force of time, space and karma

Kapha—biological water humor

Koshas—sheaths, bodies or fields around the soul

Krishna—bliss avatar of Lord Vishnu

Kriya Yoga—energetic yogic practices of pranayama, mantra and meditation

Ojas—inner power of endurance, immunity and patience

Lakshmi—Goddess of beauty, abundance and devotion

Laya—mergence, particularly into the sound current

Linga—Shiva symbol of ascending cosmic energy

Loka—plane of experience or world

Mahat—Cosmic Mind

Nada—sound vibration

Nadi—pranic channel of the subtle body

Pitta—biological fire humor

Prakasha—Shiva as pure light

Prakriti—Nature as a power of manifestation

Prana—life-force and cosmic energy

Purusha—Atman as the cosmic being

Raja Yoga—integral yoga of body, mind and spirit

Rajas—guna or quality of agitation or change

Rama—protective avatar of Vishnu

Ratri—night as a mystical and yogic symbol

Rudra—fierce or fiery form of Shiva

Sarasvati—Goddess of wisdom and art

Sat—power of being

Sattva—guna or quality of balance or endurance

Shabda—cosmic sound

Shakti—energy as a spiritual and cosmic principle

Shambhavi—Goddess as the power of perception

Shambhavi Mudra—inner fixing of the gaze

Shankara—name of Shiva and of great Vedantic teacher

Shiva—pure consciousness as the supreme principle: the destroyer/transformer among the three aspects of the cosmic lord

Soma—water or the nourishing fluidic aspect of life as a cosmic, yogic and biological principle

Sundari/Tripura Sundari—form of the Goddess governing beauty, bliss and the crown chakra

Surya—Sun or solar energy as cosmic principle

Sushumna—central channel or spine of the subtle body and chakras

Tamas—guna or quality of inertia and decay

Tantra—energetic Yoga teachings

Tapas—power of self-discipline

Tara—Goddess of inner fire of knowledge

Tejas—spiritual energy of fire

Vastu—Vedic science of directional influences

Vata—biological air humor

Vayu—wind as a cosmic principle

Vedas—mantric scriptures of the ancient seers

Vedanta—Vedic philosophy of Self-realization

Vidyut—cosmic electrical energy; also called 'tadit'

Vishnu—cosmic lord as the sustainer of the universe

Yajna—sacrifice or worship, inner sacrifice as the practice of Yoga

Yantra—geometrical concentration designs

Yoginis—Goddesses as powers of Yoga

Yoni—Shakti symbol, circular, triangular in form.

Bibliography

Abhinavagupta. PARATRISIKA VIVARANA (Jaidev Singh translation). Delhi, India: Motilal Banarsidass, 1988.

Abhinavagupta. TANTRASARA (Sanskrit only). Delhi, India:
Bani Prakashan, 1983.

Avalon, Arthur/ Sir John Woodroofe. THE SERPENT POWER.
Mineola, NY: Dover Books, 1974.

AKASHA BHAIRAVA TANTRA (Sanskrit and Hindi). Nanak Chand
Sharma, editor. Delhi, India: Motilal Banarsidass, 1980.

Ashley -Farrand, Thomas. SHAKTI MANTRAS: TAPPING INTO
THE GREAT GODDESS ENERGY WITHIN. New York City:
Ballantine Books, 2003.

Chopra, Shambhavi. YOGINI: UNFOLDING THE GODDESS
WITHIN Delhi, India: Wisdom Tree Books, 2006.

Daivarata, Brahmarshi. VAK SUDHA (Sanskrit only).

DEVI BHAGAVATAM (Sanskrit only). Varanasi, India:
Chawkhamba, 1989.

DEVI GITA (trans. by Swami Satyananda Saraswati). Napa, California: Devi Mandir, 2000.

Dikshit, Rajesh. THE DASA MAHAVIDYA (Hindi and Sanskrit).
Agra, India: Deepa Publications, 2003.

Frawley, David. TANTRIC YOGA AND THE WISDOM GOD-
DESSES. Twin Lakes, Wis.: Lotus Press 2003.

Frawley, David. YOGA AND AYURVEDA: SELF-HEALING AND
SELF-REALIZATION. Twin Lakes, Wis.: Lotus Press 1999.

Frawley, David. YOGA AND THE SACRED FIRE: SELF-REAL-
IZATION AND PLANETARY TRANSFORMATION. Twin
Lakes, Wis.: Lotus Press 2004.

Ganapati Muni. COLLECTED WORKS OF VASISHTHA KAVYA-
KANTHA GANAPATI MUNI (Sanskrit only), in eleven
volumes, edited by K. Natesan. Thiruvannamalai, India:
Sri Ramanasramam 2003–2007.

Johari, Haresh. TOOLS FOR TANTRA. Rochester, Vermont: Inner Traditions International, 1986.

Johnsen, Linda. DAUGHTERS OF THE GODDESS: THE WOMAN SAINTS OF INDIA. Saint Paul, Min.: Yes Publishers, 1994.

Johnsen, Linda. THE LOST GODDESS: RECLAIMING THE TRADITION OF THE MOTHER OF THE UNIVERSE, Saint Paul, Minn.: Yes Publishers, 2002.

Patañjali, YOGA SUTRAS. Varanasi, India: Bharatiya Vidya Prakashana, 1983, with commentaries of Vachaspati Mishra and Vijnana Bhikshu.

Ramakrishna, THE GOSPEL OF RAMAKRISHNA. Chennai, India: Sri Ramakrishna Math, 2000.

Satguru Sivaya Subramuniyaswami. DANCING WITH SHIVA. India and USA: Himalayan Academy, 1993.

Satguru Sivaya Subramuniyaswami. LOVING GANESHA. India and USA: Himalayan Academy, 1993.

Shankaracharya. SAUNDARYA LAHARI (V.K. Subramanian trans.). Delhi, India: Motilal Banarsidass, 1986.

UPANISHADS, ONE HUNDRED AND EIGHTY EIGHT (Sanskrit only). Delhi, India: Motilal Banarsidass, 1980.

VIJNANA BHAIRAVA (Commentary by Swami Lakshman Joo). Varanasi India: Indica Books, 2002.

YOGINI HRIDAYA TANTRA (Sanskrit only). Delhi, India: Motilal Banarsidass, 1980.

Index Inner Tantric Yoga

Endnotes

[1]Here the 'Antaranga Yoga' is emphasized, the Yoga of the inner limbs of Yoga, dharana, dhyana and samadhi or the Yoga of the meditative mind. Most Yoga today is only the 'Bahiranga Yoga', the Yoga of the outer limbs of Yoga, which refers to the five initial limbs of Yoga as yama, niyama, asana, pranayama and pratyahara, particularly asana. It is important to give more emphasis to the inner Yoga than the outer Yoga if we want to really practice Yoga.

[2]*Isha Upanishad,* 6–7.

[3]*Yoga Sutras* II. 44.

[4]Svadhyaya in Sanskrit also refers to studying the branch of the Vedas, adhyaya that is in one's own family.

[5]*Yoga Sutras* I.23, II.1, II.32, II.45.

[6]*Yoga Sutras* II.45.

[7]*Mundaka Upanishad* I.1.

[8]*Taittiriya Upanishad,* Shantipath.

[9]*Chandogya Upanishad* III.19.1, for example.

[10]*Isha Upanishad* 16.

[11]Note the *Bhagavad Gita* IV.24 for Brahmagni.

[12]As articulated in the *Mahabharata, Ramayana, Puranas* and *Tantras.*

[13]All the philosophical and theological issues of theism are examined in Vedic philosophies of Vedanta, Nyaya, Vaisheshika and Yoga, though Buddhism and a few Hindu sects do not recognize any Ishvara or God who has created the universe. Perhaps the most important book on Vedic theology is the *Brahma Sutras,* the main text of Vedanta.

[14]He (Ishvara) is the guru even of the ancient gurus, as he is not limited by time." *Yoga Sutras* I.26.

[15]*Yoga Sutras* I.2, for Yoga as the nirodha or calming of the mind or chitta.

[16]*Bhagavad Gita* V.24, for the attainment of Brahma Nirvana.

[17]*Kena Upanishad* I.2.

[18]Note the author's book *Ayurveda and the Mind: the Healing of Consciousness,* for an extensive examination of Ayurvedic psychology.

[19]The linga or subtle body, sukshma sharira, in Samkhya and Yoga teachings is composed of the buddhi (intelligence), ego, mind, five sense organs, five motor organs and five subtle elements.

[20]Some modern scholars have gone so far as to reduce Hindu Gods and Goddesses to sexual symbols. They would propose that a figure like Ganesha, with his head cut off by his own father Shiva, was nothing more than a manifestation of the Oedipal complex, missing his deeper yogic implications altogether. Of course, such psychological studies have been done on Christianity and Judaism as well. Freud tried to reduce the story Moses to the Oedipal complex, starting this trend. Such sexual reductionism makes us unable to understand the greater polarity of forces of which sexuality is but a manifestation. It tries to turn all spiritual and naturalistic dualities into some sort of sexual obsession, though the obsession probably dwells more in the minds of those who propose it than in the ancient texts where they see it.

[21]Prakasha Matra in Sanskrit.

[22]The *Vedas* contain many references to the worship of pillars as stambha, skambha, and dharuna. Even the term Dharma originally relates to a pillar as that which upholds all things, deriving from the root 'dri' meaning 'to uphold'.

[23]Chit-Shakti is one with Shiva, Purusha or Atman, not a principle apart. Maya is inherent in the Atman but represents a vision that moves outwardly into division and multiplicity. Prakriti arises from Maya, but contains the reflection of the Atman as the Soul in Nature. Prakriti is mainly a force of bondage through its qualities or gunas of Sattva (harmony), Rajas (agitation) and Tamas (inertia). Maya is a force of illusion through its magic creative power. Chit-Shakti, the power of consciousness, is beyond the gunas and ignorance and illusion. Once we go back to that core

Chit-Shakti, everything gets resolved into the unitary light of existence and bliss.

[24]Ganapati Muni discusses this lightning force relative to the Goddesses Indrani, Chinnamasta and Renuka, which are all related to it. Such works are found in Volume Two of the *Collected Works of Vasishtha Kavyakantha Ganapati Muni,* including Indrani Sapasati, Prachandachandi Trishati, Renuka Shatkam and Renuka Saptakam.

[25]We can use certain mantras to honor the gunas: **OM sam sattvaguṇāya namaḥ! OM ram rajoguṇāya namaḥ! OM tam tamoguṇāya namaḥ!**

[26]We can also use the mantras for these Goddesses. **Om Aim Mahāsarasvatyai namaḥ! Om Srīm Mahālakṣmyai namah! OM Krīm Mahākālyai namaḥ!**

[27]As in the Mahavidya Sutram of Volume Five of the *Collected Works of Vasishtha Kavyakantha Ganapati Muni.*

[28]Another way to work with the senses is mantra and meditation on their ruling deities. These are Vedic in nature, with the directions of space for the ears, Sun for the eye, Fire for speech, the Moon for the mind and the Wind or Vayu for Prana.

[29]Note author's *Yoga and Ayurveda,* Chapter 9, for more information on the five pranas.

[30]*Yoga Sutras.* I.2.

[31]*Yoga Sutras.* IV.34. svarupapratista va chiti Shakti.

[32]The author has addressed this approach in *Yoga for Your Type.*

[33]For example, Bhastrika pranayama has its characteristic heating energy on the mind and senses. It is often used to stimulate the Kundalini. Shitali has a characteristic cooling energy.

[34]Note the *Upanishads* for this teaching, *Brihadaranyaka Upanishad* I.4.2.

[35]These are called *rasa, virya, vipaka* and *prabhava* in Sanskrit.

[36]The author's book along with Dr. Vasant Lad, the *Yoga of Herbs,*

explains these herbal energetics and how to combine them, which is the art of herbal yoga.

[37]Note author's Tantric *Yoga and the Wisdom Goddesses: Spiritual Secrets of Ayurveda*: Ojas, pp. 215–219.

[38]Note author's *Tantric Yoga and the Wisdom Goddesses* for a discussion of Prana, Tejas and Ojas.

[39]This small space is called *dahara akasha* in Sanskrit as in the *Chandogya Upanishad,* Chapter VIII.

[40]What is called *Atma-vichara* in Sanskrit, such as in the teachings of Ramana Maharashi.

[41]The practice of Yoga arose as the inner counterpart of the Vedic sacrifice. Note the fourth chapter of the *Bhagavad Gita* for a description of yogic practices as internal sacrifices.

[42]*Mundaka Upanishad* II.4.

[43]*Durga Sukta* of the *Mahanarayana Upanishad, Taittiriya Aranyaka* IV.10.2.

[44]*Sri Sukta. Rig-Veda Parisisthani* or Appendix.

[45]The *satyakama* of the *Upanishads, Chandogya Upanishad* VIII.31.

[46]This is called *Tarpaka Kapha* in Ayurvedic medicine, one of the five forms of Kapha governing the lubrication of the brain and nervous system.

[47]Ganapati Muni was of this opinion and said Kundalini was the power of the Jivatman.

[48]Bhairavi is also one of the Ten Great Goddesses or Dasha Mahavidya. Note author's *Tantric Yoga and the Wisdom Goddesses* in this regard.

[49]*Svetasvatara Upanishad* II.1.

[50]These are the four states of speech in yogic and Tantric thought of *Vaikhari, Madhyama, Pashyanti* and *Para.*

[51]Note the author's book, *Yoga and the Sacred Fire,* for more information on this topic of the soul and fire.

[52]Bhastrika and Kapalabhati pranayamas are particularly strong for this purpose, but require much caution in their usage.

[53]The dragon or *Ahi-vrtra* symbolizes the ego forces or unawakened Kundalini that keeps us bound to the realm of ignorance and suffering.

[54]In the Tantric Mantra Purusha or person of sound, the sound-I corresponds to the right eye and the sound-Ī to the left eye. Note *Yoga and Ayurveda* Chapter 17 for its chapter on the Mantra Purusha.

[55]Notably the famous *Rudram* chant from the *Krishna Yajur Veda*.

[56]So'ham or Hamsa work well as mantras with full nostril breathing, like the Ujjayi breath. They can also be used with forceful full nostril breathing as with Bhastrika and Kapalabhati.

[57]They are called antahstha or intermediate sounds in Sanskrit.

[58]In the Mantra Purusha or cosmic being of sound, the semi-vowels and sibilants correspond to the tissues and energies of the body. So their usage energizes the life in the representational form of the deity. **Yam** relates to plasma, **Ram** to blood, **Lam** to muscle, **Vam** to fat, **Śam** to bone, **Ṣam** to nerve, **Sam** to reproductive tissue, **Ham** to Prana and **Kṣam** to mind.

[59]The Gayatri Mantra can be used in this regard as well.

[60]A longer Shiva mantra for Shiva as the Lord of Yogis is: **Om Haum Jūm Saḥ Shivaya Yogeśvarāya Namaḥ!**

[61]Abhinavagupta's *Tantra Sara VI.* Masodaya section, for example.

[62]This process is also symbolized astrologically. The half of the zodiac from 0 Aquarius to 0 Leo or the signs from Aquarius to Cancer, indicate the lunar ascent. The half of the zodiac from 0 Leo to 0 Aquarius or the signs from Leo to Capricorn, indicate the solar descent. These mark the two halves of the year.

[63]Such meters are called Gayatri, trishtubh, jagati and others, which are modulated relative to the rishi who composes the Vedic hymn and the deity or Devata to which it is addressed.

[64]*Chandogya Upanishad*, III.14.1.

[65]*Svetesvatara Upanishad*, Devatma Shakti.

[66]*Gods, Sages and Kings* (Lotus Press), *In Search of the Cradle of*

Civilization (Quest Books), *Hidden Horizons: Unearthing 10,000 Years of Indian Culture* (Swaminarayan Publications, BAPS).

[67]For example, N.S. Rajaram, Subhash Kak, Michel Danino, B.B. Lal, Shivaji Singh, Kalyanaraman and Vishal Agarwal.

[68]Such practices are found mainly in the *Atharva Veda*. It is not so much a question of these being outside the Vedic tradition as being non-sattvic in nature and so sometimes rejected as unspiritual.

[69]For example, the bija **Krīm** for action or Kriya is hidden the Vedic root 'kri' meaning to do.

[70]The mantra **Īm** is the most common mantric interjection in the *Rig-Veda,* being replaced by **OM** in the *Yajur-Veda,* as explained by Brahmarshi Daivarata in his *Vak Sudha.* The *Sama-Veda* has various short sounds or bijas that it interjects into its tonalities. The *Upanishads* explain **OM** in great detail but use many other seed syllables and short word forms for its teachings.

[71]A good text in this regard is *Paratrisika Vivarana* of Abhinavagupta, for which there is a good modern translation and commentary by Jaideva Singh, who has done many other important such books on Kashmir Shaivism and Tantra.

[72]*Chandogya Upanishad* II.22.3.

[73]*Aitareya Aranyaka* II.3.8.20.

[74]*Aitareya Aranyaka* III.2.1.7. Prana ushmarupam. Also II.2.4.12.

[75]The writings of Ganapati Muni contain a number of references to the unity of Indra and Shiva, notably his *Indreshvarabheda Sutra.* Unfortunately, little of this has yet been translated from the Sanskrit.

About the Author

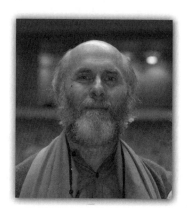

Dr. David Frawley (Pandit Vamadeva Shastri) is one of the few westerners ever regarded in India as an authentic Vedacharya, or Vedic teacher, where he has taught and lectured throughout the country. Over the last thirty years, he has written thirty books on Yoga, Ayurveda, Vedic astrology, Vedanta and the Vedas, which have been translated into fifteen languages worldwide and are regarded as authoritative texts in their fields. He has conducted a special study of Vedic and Tantric texts in the original Sanskrit, following the teachings of the great disciple of Ramana Maharshi, Ganapati Muni, which is the basis of the current book.

Vamadeva conducts training programs in the United States, Europe, South America and India through a broad network of affiliated organizations. The goal of his work is to promote the main branches of Vedic and yogic knowledge in a comprehensive and integral manner for the planetary age. He is the director of the American Institute of Vedic Studies in Santa Fe, New Mexico.

American Institute of Vedic Studies
PO Box 8357, Santa Fe NM 87504-8357
David Frawley (Vamadeva Shastri), Director
Web: www.vedanet.com

The American Institute of Vedic Studies is an educational center devoted to the greater systems of Vedic and yogic knowledge. It teaches related aspects of Vedic Science including Ayurveda, Vedic Astrology, Yoga and Vedanta with a special reference to their background in the Vedas. It offers extensive articles, books, courses and training programs and is engaged in several important research projects. It is connected to many organizations worldwide and offers a special resource guide.

Ayurvedic Healing Distance Learning Program in Ayurvedic Medicine

This comprehensive program covers all the main aspects of Ayurvedic theory and practice. It is not just an introduction to Ayurveda but a full training program on Ayurveda in all of its branches, including the Ayurvedic view of body and mind, the disease process and diagnosis, and Ayurvedic treatment through diet, herbs, sensory therapies, Yoga and meditation.

The goal of the course is to provide students a foundation for becoming Ayurvedic practitioners. Since 1988 over five thousand people worldwide have taken the course, which has also been used as textbook material for two year Ayurveda colleges in the West.

Advanced Yoga and Ayurveda Distance Learning Program

This unique course teaches the healing and transformational approaches of both Yoga and Ayurveda. It is not simply an asana course but shows the therapeutic application of all eight limbs of Yoga, including pranayama, pratyahara, mantra and meditation. It contains a complete study of the Yoga Sutras from an Ayurvedic angle. It introduces Ayurvedic Yoga and its Vedic equivalents (Vedic Yoga). It brings in the perspective of Tantra relative to the energetics of the subtle body and the use of mantras.

The course aims at providing the student with the foundation for an integrated Yoga-Ayurveda therapy on physical, psychological and spiritual levels, considering the greater Yoga tradition.

Vedic Astrology and Ayurveda Distance Learning Program

This comprehensive training program explains Vedic astrology in clear and modern terms, providing practical insights how to use and adapt the system for the contemporary student.

The course is unique in that it teaches Vedic astrology with a special reference to Ayurveda medicine. This distinguishes it from other introductory courses on Vedic astrology in which the Ayurvedic component is minor. The course is of special interest to Ayurvedic students and for those looking to specialize in medical astrology.